SCLERODERMA

SYMPTOMS, DIAGNOSIS AND TREATMENT

IMMUNOLOGY AND IMMUNE SYSTEM DISORDERS

Additional books in this series can be found on Nova's website under the Series tab.

Additional e-books in this series can be found on Nova's website under the e-book tab.

DERMATOLOGY – LABORATORY AND CLINICAL RESEARCH

Additional books in this series can be found on Nova's website under the Series tab.

Additional e-books in this series can be found on Nova's website under the e-book tab.

IMMUNOLOGY AND IMMUNE SYSTEM DISORDERS

SCLERODERMA

SYMPTOMS, DIAGNOSIS AND TREATMENT

ROMAIN DE WINTER
EDITOR

New York

Copyright © 2013 by Nova Science Publishers, Inc.

For permission to use material from this book please contact us:
Telephone 631-231-7269; Fax 631-231-8175
Web Site: http://www.novapublishers.com

NOTICE TO THE READER

Additional color graphics may be available in the e-book version of this book.

Library of Congress Cataloging-in-Publication Data

ISBN: 978-1-62618-802-0

LCCN: 2013937397

Published by Nova Science Publishers, Inc. † New York

Contents

Preface

Systemic sclerosis or scleroderma is an autoimmune disease characterized by widespread microangiopathy, immune system alterations and fibrosis of the skin and internal organs. This book presents current research in the study of the symptoms, diagnosis and treatment of scleroderma. Topics discussed include the identification and treatment of the pulmonary manifestations of systemic sclerosis; interstitial lung disease in systemic sclerosis; nailfold capillaroscopy and early diagnosis of systemic sclerosis; localized scleroderma; evaluation of a new CENPB epitope array for systemic sclerosis-associated centromere autoantibodies; and iloprost in the treatment of Raynaud phenomenon secondary to scleroderma.

Chapter I – Over 80% of patients with Systemic Sclerosis (SSc) have associated lung involvement. Pulmonary manifestations consist of chronic aspiration, interstitial lung disease (ILD) and pulmonary hypertension (PH), with the latter two conditions being the most common causes of mortality. Individuals with ILD and PH typically first present with dyspnea on exertion which must be differentiated from dyspnea caused by cardiac involvement, myositis from overlap syndromes and deconditioning. As a result, identifying the etiology of dyspnea in patients with this disease is complicated and can require extensive testing. Treatment options for ILD are limited and only cyclophosphamide has been shown to have efficacy in clinical trials, but other therapies such as mycophenolate, rituximab, and stem cell transplant are under investigation. PH treatment is based on the etiology of the elevated pulmonary pressures, which can arise from either hypoxic vasoconstriction from ILD, pulmonary venous hypertension from cardiac involvement, or direct involvement of the pulmonary vasculature – pulmonary arterial hypertension (PAH). Treatment of PAH in SSc is similar to treatment of PAH in other conditions, and involves endothelin receptor antagonists, phosphodiesterase-5 inhibitors, and prostacyclin analogs. For both ILD and PAH, lung trans-plantation may be an option in cases where medical therapy is ineffective.

Chapter II – Systemic sclerosis or scleroderma (SSc) is an autoimmune disease characterized by a widespread microangiopathy, immune system alterations and fibrosis of the skin and internal organs. Lung involvement is a frequent complication and interstitial lung disease (ILD) represents a leading cause of morbidity and mortality in SSc patients. Unlike idiopathic ILD, SSc-ILD corresponds to non-specific interstitial pneumonia (NSIP) in most cases, whereas usual interstitial pneumonia (UIP) is less frequently encountered. Therefore, the prognosis of SSc-ILD is better than that for idiopathic ILD. However, in a small number of cases, it may progress rapidly to end-stage respiratory insufficiency. Thoracic high-resolution computed tomography (HRCT), pulmonary function tests (PFT) including carbon monoxide diffusing capacity (DLCO) and 6-minute walk (6MWT) test with measurement of oxygen saturation are essential at the time of diagnosis of SSc. Generally, a lung biopsy is not needed in patients with SSc-ILD, except in the case of a discrepancy between clinical manifestations and HRCT findings. Treatment of ILD remains disappointing although many promising therapies are emerging. Cyclophosphamide (CYC), which has been used for 20 years, has recently been evaluated in two prospective randomized studies that failed to demonstrate a major benefit for lung function. Mycophenolate mofetil, azathioprine and rituximab are as alternatives to CYC. Promising cellular and molecular targeted anti-fibrotic therapeutic options have emerged. Lung transplantation can be proposed in the absence of other major organ involvement.

Chapter III – Nailfold capillaroscopy is an essential imaging technique and the best method to analyse microvascular abnormalities in autoimmune rheumatic diseases. Capillary microscopy seems to be a useful tool for early selection of those patients who are potentially candidates for developing scleroderma spectrum disorders, especially systemic sclerosis (SSc). Architectural disorganization, giant capillaries, haemorrhages, loss of capillaries, angiogenesis and avascular areas characterize >90% of patients with overt SSc. The term "SSc pattern" includes, all together, these sequential capillaroscopic changes typical to the microvascular involvement in SSc. Three different patterns identified within the "SSc pattern"-early, active and late. Several different laboratory variables (serum E-selectin, serum tissue kallikrein, plasma endothelin 1, homocystein, urinary metabolites of F2-isoprostanes, serum anti-endothelial cell antibodies, antitopoisomerase I antibodies, anticentromere antibodies, anti-CENP-B, anti Th/To antibodies and anti-RNAP III) and clinical manifestations in SSc (peripheral vascular, skin, and lung involvement) have been shown to be associated with different pattern of capillary abnormality, providing further insights into disease pathogenesis.

Chapter IV – Scleroderma is a rare fibrosing disorder of the skin and underlying tissues characterized by skin thickening and hardening due to an increased collagen density. The approximate incidence varies according to race, but is approximately 0.4-2.7 per 100 000 persons. Its exact pathogenesis is still unknown, but several triggering factors in genetically predisposed individuals might lead to release of pro-inflammatory cytokines, which results in dysregulation of connective tissue metabolism and ultimately to fibrosis. Scleroderma can be divided into localized scleroderma or morphea, which is the focus of this chapter, and systemic scleroderma (SSc). Several clinical forms of localized scleroderma exist including morphea en plaque, generalized morphea, guttate morphea, nodular morphea, subcutaneous morphea and linear scleroderma. Treatment depends on the type; circumscribed forms may benefit topical treatment, while generalized or linear lesions would require systemic treatment. Although localized scleroderma has a good prognosis in general, some clinical subtypes of the disease can be very deforming and irreversibly disabling, especially when affecting the extremities or the face.

Chapter V – Systemic sclerosis (SSc) is a heterogeneous autoimmune disorder characterized by the presence of antinuclear autoantibodies (ANA). The ANA classically detected in SSc include anticentromere antibodies (ACA) which are positive in 50-60% of the patients. The centromere protein CENPB is a major autoantigen reactive with SSc sera showing a typical immunofluorescence staining pattern. Previously, epitopes on CENPB were identified in the N-terminal (Nt) and C-terminal (Ct) domains of the autoantigen and this form the rationale for an specific multi-parallel detection of CENPB epitopes in SSc. Using recombinant CENPB Nt and Ct domains the Author developed a new fluorescent array immunoassay for ACA detection in SSc patients. 81 sera from patients with SSc, SLE and normal controls were evaluated. From 27 ACA positive sera tested, 25 were CENPB positive by ECL blot techniques. Among them our fluorescent array showed 23 Nt-CENPB and 12 Ct-CENPB positives. 10 Ct-CENPB were also Nt-CENPB positive by the array assay. 13 Nt-CENPB were Ct-CENPB negative and only 2 Ct-CENPB positive sera were Nt-CENPB negative. This result shows a prevalence of Nt-CENPB epitope over Ct-CENPB in ACA positive SSc patients. The CENPB fluorescent array developed has good agreement with conventional techniques for selected ACA and has the advantage of multi-parallel detection of CENPB autoepitopes in SSc.

Chapter VI – Objective: To highlight iloprost as a choice drug in the Raynaud phenomenon secondary to systemic sclerosis, and to forewarn people about the development of a possible paradoxical reaction when repeated intravenous cycles are received. Background: Raynaud phenomenon occurs in more than 90% of patients with systemic sclerosis. Digital arteries and precapillary arterioles show marked fibrosis of the intima and luminal narrowing, being associated with platelet activation and abnormal vascular reactivity. Iloprost is a prostacyclin analog with vasodilating and platelet inhibitory effects, providing increased blood flow. Discussion: The intravenous prostanoids (particularly short-term intravenous infusions of iloprost) have proved to be efficacious in healing digital ulcers and severe Raynaud phenomenon in patients with systemic sclerosis (strength of European League against Rheumatism Scleroderma Trials and Research group- EUSTAR- recommendation A). However, paradoxical reaction of Raynaud phenomenon has been reported in a patient with diffuse cutaneous systemic sclerosis, associated with repeated administration and increased infusion rate of iloprost (probable relationship according to Naranjo probability scale). Conclusion: Iloprost in treatment of patients with Raynaud phenomenon could be involved in a paradoxical reaction. Physicians should be aware of this adverse event and patients should be monitored (tolerance and clinical response).

In: Scleroderma   ISBN: 978-1-62618-802-0
Editor: Romain De Winter   © 2013 Nova Science Publishers, Inc.

Chapter I

Identification and Treatment of the Pulmonary Manifestations of Systemic Sclerosis

Todd Davidyock* and Arthur C. Theodore
Boston University School of Medicine, Boston, MA

Abstract

Over 80% of patients with Systemic Sclerosis (SSc) have associated lung involvement. Pulmonary manifestations consist of chronic aspiration, interstitial lung disease (ILD) and pulmonary hypertension (PH), with the latter two conditions being the most common causes of mortality. Individuals with ILD and PH typically first present with dyspnea on exertion which must be differentiated from dyspnea caused by cardiac involvement, myositis from overlap syndromes and decon-ditioning. As a result, identifying the etiology of dyspnea in patients with this disease is complicated and can require extensive testing. Treatment options for ILD are limited and only cyclophosphamide has been shown to have efficacy in clinical trials, but other therapies such as myco-phenolate, rituximab, and stem cell transplant are under investigation. PH treatment is based on the etiology of the elevated pulmonary pressures, which can arise from either hypoxic vasoconstriction from ILD,

---

* Email: todavidy@bu.edu.

pulmonary venous hypertension from cardiac involvement, or direct involvement of the pulmonary vasculature – pulmonary arterial hypertension (PAH). Treatment of PAH in SSc is similar to treatment of PAH in other conditions, and involves endothelin receptor antagonists, phosphodiesterase-5 inhibitors, and prostacyclin analogs. For both ILD and PAH, lung transplantation may be an option in cases where medical therapy is ineffective.

Introduction

Systemic sclerosis (SSc) is a complex, autoimmune disease charac-terized by multi-organ fibrosis, vasculopathy and various autoantibodies. (Gabrielli, Avvedimento et al. 2009) It has a prevalence of 233-277 cases per million people with an estimated 75,000-100,000 affected individuals in the United States. (Nikpour, Stevens et al. 2010, Mayes, Lacey et al. 2003) There are 2 major sub-classifications of the disease, limited and diffuse, based upon the extent of skin involvement, with limited disease usually only confined to the skin of the face, neck, and distal portion of the arms beyond the elbows. Cardiopulmonary complications are the leading cause of morbidity and mortality among individuals with either limited or diffuse SSc. (Steen, Medsger 2007)

Over 80% of individuals with SSc develop lung involvement(Ferri, Valentini et al. 2002) primarily consisting of ILD and PH. (Steen, Medsger 2007) Interstitial lung disease (ILD) can manifest in various patterns, with non-specific interstitial pneumonia (NSIP) being the most common pattern seen on high resolution computed tomography (HRCT). (Bouros, Wells et al. 2002, Kim, Yoo et al. 2002, Fischer, Swigris et al. 2008) Pulmonary hypertension (PH) can result from direct involvement of the pulmonary vasculature - PAH, secondary to cardiac involvement - pulmonary venous hypertension (PVH), or as a consequence of hypoxic vasoconstriction from advanced ILD. Less commonly, individuals may develop pulmonary complications from aspiration related to esophageal dysmotility, and can also develop pleural effusions, pneumothoraces, bronchiectasis, and lung cancer.

Individuals with lung involvement typically first present with shortness of breath. Determining the etiology of the primary limitation in SSc is complicated by the myriad pathologic states that can lead to dyspnea, which include diseases of the cardiopulmonary system noted above, as well as myositis in overlap syndromes and deconditioning from chronic disease. An extensive work-up including pulmonary function testing, radiography, echocardiography, bronchoscopy, and biopsy, may be necessary to elucidate the exact cause. This review will focus on the diagnostic work-up and management of the pulmonary complications in SSc, specifically focusing on ILD and PAH, the two most common conditions.

Epidemiology

ILD and PAH account for 60% of SSc related deaths. (Steen, Medsger 2007) Approximately 40% of individuals with SSc develop ILD(Hassoun 2011) which is more commonly associated with the diffuse cutaneous form. (Ostojic, Damjanov 2006) A large cohort showed it is also associated with African American ethnicity, high skin score, serum creatinine and creatinine phosphokinase values, hypothyroidism, and electrocardiography and echocardiography defined cardiac involvement. (McNearney, Reveille et al. 2007) The same cohort showed presence of anti-centromere antibodies had a protective effect. Severe ILD in SSc, defined as a forced vital capacity <55% on pulmonary function testing, has a survival rate of 30% at 9 years. (Steen, Medsger 2000)

PAH, defined as a mean pulmonary artery pressure greater than 25 mm Hg with a pulmonary artery occlusive pressure less than 15 mm Hg on right heart catheterization,(McLaughlin, Archer et al. 2009) is found in 8-12% of the SSc population. (York, Farber 2011) It is generally thought to occur in the later stages of disease in the limited cutaneous form of SSc,(Medsger 2003) though it can still occur frequently in diffuse cutaneous SSc. (Mukerjee, St George et al. 2003, MacGregor, Canavan et al. 2001) PAH has been found to be associated with increased numbers of telangiectasias, reduced capillary nailfold density, anti-centromere antibodies, anti-topoisomerase antibodies, male sex, underlying pulmonary fibrosis, and Raynaud's phenomenon of greater than 3 years' duration. (York, Farber 2011) Individuals with SSc associated PAH also tend to have increased plasma levels of N-terminal probrain natriuretic peptide (N-T proBNP). (Schioppo, Artusi et al. 2012) A recent, large study showed that subjects with PAH had a survival rate of approximately 56% at 3 years. (Hachulla, Carpentier et al. 2009).

Diagnosis

Clinical Symptoms and Signs

The clinical history can be limited in its utility for discerning significant pulmonary involvement, as individuals with SSc often report dyspnea on exertion as a symptom. This can be caused both by intrinsic cardiopulmonary disease, such as ILD and PAH, as well as other manifestations of SSc, such as myositis in overlap syndromes or deconditioning from chronic disease. A dry cough, however, is a common symptom of ILD, and has been found to be associated with the extent of fibrosis in SSc. (Theodore, Tseng et al. 2012) Individuals with advanced PAH may report palpitations from arrhythmias, or syncopal episodes with activity.

The lung exam in ILD may be normal, or may show fine, basilar, "Velcro"-like inspiratory crackles. (Alton, Turner-Warwick 1988) Cardiopulmonary physical exam findings in PAH depend on the severity of disease, but would be consistent with right ventricular overload and include an increased P2, murmur of tricuspid regurgitation, right sided S4, right ventricular heave, elevated jugular venous distension, and peripheral edema. (McLaughlin, Archer et al. 2009) In both ILD and PAH, individuals may manifest resting hypoxemia, or become hypoxemic on ambulation.

Radiography and High Resolution Commuted Tomography

SSc associated ILD manifests on plain chest radiographs as ground-glass opacification (GGO) with a superimposed reticular pattern. (Wells, Steen et al. 2009) (Table 1) Advanced disease may show traction bronchiectasis and honey combing. (Strollo, Goldin 2010) Unfortunately, chest radiography is insensitive for early ILD with only a small fraction of chest x-rays showing evidence of increased interstitial markings. (Steele, Hudson et al. 2012) Plain chest radiography is less useful in identifying the presence of PAH. Chest x-rays can be normal, or may show decreased peripheral lung markings, prominent pulmonary arteries, or right ventricular enlargement. (McLaughlin, Archer et al. 2009)

HRCT is much more sensitive for identifying interstitial changes of the pulmonary parenchyma associated with SSc. (Desai, Veeraraghavan et al. 2004, Muller, Miller 1990, Pignone, Matucci-Cerinic et al. 1992,

Schurawitzki, Stiglbauer et al. 1990, Strickland, Strickland 1988) The earliest manifestations are subpleural septal thickening alone or associated with GGO. (Le Pavec, Launay et al. 2011) (Figure 1) GGO may be diffuse or localized and occur both without (pure GGO) and with (mixed GGO) fibrotic changes. Pathologically, the pattern is classically described as fibrotic non-specific interstitial pneumonitis (NSIP) and is found most commonly. (Kim, Yoo et al. 2002, Bouros, Wells et al. 2002, Fischer, Swigris et al. 2008)

Table 1. Expected results for the major diagnostic tests for interstitial lung disease and pulmonary arterial hypertension in scleroderma

	Interstitial Lung Disease	Pulmonary Arterial Hypertension
Chest X-Ray	*Early:* GGO Reticular Markings *Late:* Traction bronchiectasis Honeycombing	Decreased peripheral lung markings Prominent main PA Enlarged RV
High Resolution CT	*Early:* Bilateral, lower lobe, subpleural GGO Septal thickening *Later:* Diffuse GGO[a] Traction Bronchiectasis[b] Honeycombing[b]	Increased main PA diameter
Pulmonary Function Testing	Decreased FVC Decreased DLCO	Decreased DLCO
Echocardiography	Increased peak systolic PA pressure[*]	Increased peak systolic PA pressure *Late:* Tricuspid regurgitation RV Dilatation
Right Heart Catheterization	Increased mean PA pressure[*] Normal wedge pressure	Increased mean PA pressure Normal wedge pressure
Bronchoalveolar Lavage	Increased neutrophils and eosinophils	N/A
Lung Biopsy	NSIP UIP	Pulmonary artery intimal thickening Decreased pulmonary artery lumen diameter

a:Typically with non-specific interstitial pneumonia phenotype; b: Typically with usual interstitial pneumonia phenotype.

*: if secondary pulmonary hypertension also present.

PA: pulmonary artery, RV: right ventricle, GGO: ground glass opacities, FVC: forced vital capacity, DLCO: Diffusion capacity, NSIP: non-specific interstitial pneumonia, UIP: usual interstitial pneumonitis.

However, both cellular and mixed NSIP and usual interstitial pneumonitis (UIP) have been described with UIP most commonly associated with areas of honeycombing. (Kim, Yoo et al. 2002, Goldin, Lynch et al. 2008, Strollo, Goldin 2010).

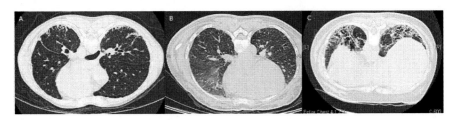

Figure 1. High resolution CT images of different presentations of interstitial lung disease in scleroderma. A: Mild basilar, subpleural fibrosis. B: Pure ground glass with only minimal fibrosis. C: Severe basilar fibrosis and honeycombing.

HRCT is potentially more useful than plain radiography for identifying signs of PAH, with some studies showing that an increased diameter of the main pulmonary artery predicts the presence of PH. (Haimovici, Trotman-Dickenson et al. 1997, Edwards, Bull et al. 1998, Kuriyama, Gamsu et al. 1984). Extensive fibrosis on HRCT also correlates well with increased mean pulmonary artery pressures in individuals with SSc associated ILD. (Pandey, Wilcox et al. 2010).

Pulmonary Function Testing

Pulmonary function testing involves dynamic measurements of inspiratory and expiratory pulmonary flows, as well as assessments of lung volumes through plethysmography and gas exchange using the diffusion of carbon monoxide (DLCO). (Behr, Furst 2008) Restrictive lung disease is evidenced by a decreased forced vital capacity (FVC) less than 80% and a preserved ratio of the forced expiratory volume in 1 second (FEV1) to FVC (FEV1/FVC greater than lower limit of normal predicted). A low DLCO provides evidence of a diffusion abnormality, which is related to involvement of the pulmonary parenchyma consistent with destruction of alveolar-capillary units from fibrosis or vasculopathy.

As much as 40% of individuals with SSc will have at least a moderate decrease in the forced vital capacity (FVC ≤ 75% predicted) suggesting restriction from ILD. (Steen, Conte et al. 1994) However, gas exchange derangements evidenced by a reduced DLCO are the earliest sign of SSc involvement of the cardiopulmonary system,(Wells, Hansell et al. 1997) and may be present in up to 70% of individuals with SSc. (Le Pavec, Launay et al. 2011) An isolated low DLCO (< 55% predicted) with a normal FVC suggests the presence of PAH, though it may also be a sign of subclinical ILD. (Steen, Graham et al. 1992) Reduction in DLCO correlates with severity of disease for both ILD and PAH. (Steen, Graham et al. 1992, Wells, Hansell et al. 1997)

Echocardiography and Right Heart Catheterization

Right heart catheterization, which allows for the measurement of right sided heart and pulmonary pressures and cardiac output, as well as an approximation of left sided diastolic filling pressure, is currently the gold standard for identifying the presence of PH. (McLaughlin, Archer et al. 2009) A resting mean pulmonary artery pressure above 25 mm Hg defines PH and can result from direct involvement of the pulmonary arteries, hypoxic vasoconstriction or from destruction related to ILD. A similar increase in mean pulmonary artery pressure is seen with left sided cardiac involvement, but the pulmonary artery occlusive pressure, or wedge pressure, is greater than or equal to 15 mm Hg in these cases.

Determining the primary cause of PH in SSc can be challenging due to the myriad etiologic pathways. PAH and PH secondary to hypoxic vasoconstriction from ILD will both have elevated mean pulmonary artery pressures with a wedge pressure less than 15 mm Hg. PH secondary to ILD is generally thought to have more modest elevations of the mean pulmonary artery pressure (25-35 mm Hg), and would be expected to have associated signs of restrictive lung disease (i.e. either FVC or total lung capacity (TLC) less than 60%) on pulmonary function testing. (York, Farber 2011) In some individuals, there may be involvement of both the pulmonary vasculature and the parenchyma leading to a combined effect, which can only be deduced clinically.

Since right heart catheterization is an invasive procedure, attempts have been made to look for less invasive means of identifying elevations of pressures in the pulmonary circulation. In addition to pulmonary function testing, Doppler echocardiography is frequently used as a screening tool. Measurement of the tricuspid regurgitant jet (TRJ) provides an estimation of the peak systolic pulmonary artery pressure and evidence for the presence of PH. (Galie, Hoeper et al. 2009) The European Society of Cardiology/European

Respiratory Society provides criteria for the utility of the TRJ measurement. Individuals with TRJ values less than 2.8 m/s, the equivalent of a pulmonary artery systolic pressure less than 36 mm Hg, are unlikely to have PH on right heart catheterization. Values of TRJ greater than 3.4 m/s, or a pulmonary artery systolic pressure greater than 50 mm Hg, are suggestive of PH, and individuals with these measurements should undergo right heart catheterization. It is reasonable to evaluate individuals who are symptomatic from a pulmonary perspective with echocardiography prior to performing right heart catheterization, since this can potentially prevent some patients from undergoing the more invasive procedure.

Bronchoalveolar Lavage and Lung Biopsy

Bronchoalveolar lavage (BAL) is a technique used during bronchoscopy to evaluate the cellular contents of the lower respiratory tract and can potentially aide in the diagnosis of SSc associated ILD. (Kowal-Bielecka, Kowal et al. 2010) In samples from normal lung, the BAL analysis reveals primarily macrophages (80-90% of cellular components) with low numbers of neutrophils and lymphoctyes. (Heron, Grutters et al. 2012) Over 50% of individuals with SSc will show an abnormal BAL with the primary difference being an increased number of neutrophils or, less commonly, eosinophils, (Silver, Metcalf et al. 1984) even in the absence of overt clinical symptoms. (Silver, Miller et al. 1990) An abnormal BAL correlates with worse lung function as evidenced by a lower DLCO. (Silver, Miller et al. 1990) BAL also may correlate with the presence and/or severity of ILD on HRCT, (Kowal-Bielecka, Kowal et al. 2010) though BAL neutrophilia can be present in the absence of any radiographic changes. (Harrison, McAnulty et al. 1990).

Although surgical lung biopsy is not always necessary to make a clinical diagnosis in SSc, it can provide confirmation of the underlying histopathology present in ILD. (American Thoracic Society, European Respiratory Society 2002) The biopsy may be most helpful though with lung findings suggesting a disease process other than that expected from SSc. (Le Pavec, Launay et al. 2011) If a biopsy is to be taken, it is recommended to target peripheral lung tissue, since the subpleural areas are most commonly affected. (Muller, Miller et al. 1986) Patterns on HRCT generally correlate well with biopsy specimen findings. (Wells, Hansell et al. 1993) As noted above, the most commonly found pathology is NSIP, and is often found when HRCT shows isolated ground glass opacities. (Fischer, Swigris et al. 2008) A reticular pattern on

HRCT is more likely to show a pathologic pattern of fibrosis on biopsy consistent with UIP. (Fischer, Swigris et al. 2008, Wells, Hansell et al. 1993) Evidence of PH, including intimal thickening of pulmonary arteries resulting in decreased lumen size, can also be seen on biopsy. (al-Sabbagh, Steen et al. 1989)

Treatment

Interstitial Lung Disease

Although the mechanism for the pathogenesis of ILD in SSc is still not completely understood, it is thought to most likely result from parenchymal injury initially manifesting as inflammation and eventually evolving into fibrosis. (Hassoun 2011, Katsumoto, Whitfield et al. 2011) Since the fibrotic changes are irreversible, the focus of treatment is reduction of inflammation with immunosuppressants.

Historically, treatment has included regimens consisting of corticosteroids alone, D-penicillamine, methotrexate, relaxin, interferon-alpha and various other medications. Research has shown, however, that these medications are not likely to be beneficial due to either being ineffective or having too many adverse effects. (Teixeira, Mouthon et al. 2008, Clements, Furst et al. 1999, van den Hoogen, Boerbooms et al. 1996, Pope, Bellamy et al. 2001, Khanna, Clements et al. 2009, Black, Silman et al. 1999)

The failure of these agents to provide benefit has led to the investigation of cyclophosphamide as a therapeutic agent. Unfortunately, this too can have significant toxicity, and new regimens are being investigated that still have yet to be proven to be effective.

As a result, initiation of treatment at the current time must involve weighing the risks and benefits for each patient. Treatment is generally recommended though in patients who report some degree of pulmonary limitation in the context of other diagnostic tests suggestive of active lung disease, either reduced or worsening FVC on pulmonary function testing or GGO on HRCT, and have no contraindications to treatment. (Le Pavec, Launay et al. 2011) Contraindications to using immunosuppressant therapy include active or suspected infections, pregnancy, breastfeeding, or neutropenia.

Cyclophosphamide

Cyclophosphamide is a nitrogen mustard alkylating agent that directly effects bone marrow precursors and mature lymphocytes resulting in decreased numbers of T and B cells and a reduced CD4:CD8 T cell ratio. (Manno, Boin 2010) It is used in chemotherapeutic regimens and as an immunosuppressive agent for treatment of autoimmune diseases, because of its anti-inflammatory effects. There have been multiple uncontrolled case series reporting its benefits in the treatment of SSc associated ILD. (Le Pavec, Launay et al. 2011) More recently, there have been two prospective studies that have helped to further clarify its utility in individuals with signs of active pulmonary disease. (Tashkin, Elashoff et al. 2006, Hoyles, Ellis et al. 2006).

The largest prospective study, the SSc Lung Study (SLS-1), was a multi-center, double-blind, randomized, placebo-controlled study, which included 158 patients with SSc, evidence of active alveolitis on BAL or HRCT, signs of lung impairment on pulmonary function testing, and dyspnea on clinical history. (Tashkin, Elashoff et al. 2006) Subjects were randomized to treatment with daily oral cyclophosphamide (up to 2 mg/kg total dose) or matching placebo for 1 year, with a planned additional year of follow-up. Subjects were also allowed to be on prednisone during the trial period as long as the dose was less than 10 mg daily. After 12 months, subjects in the cyclophosphamide group had a small but significant difference in the mean FVC percent predicted (2.53%, 95% confidence interval 0.28-4.79%). A follow-up study looking at the additional 12 months of untreated time showed that the benefits persisted for up to 6 months of this period, but then ultimately dissipated at the end of treatment, except for a sustained effect on dyspnea. (Tashkin, Elashoff et al. 2007)

A second group conducted a smaller, multi-center, double-blinded, randomized, placebo-controlled trial evaluating treatment with monthly, intravenous cyclophosphamide (mean dose 600 mg/m^2) and alternate day prednisolone for 6 months followed by 6 months of azathioprine (2.5 mg/kg day, maximum 200 mg/day). (Hoyles, Ellis et al. 2006) A total of 45 subjects who had SSc and evidence of pulmonary fibrosis by HRCT or lung biopsy underwent the protocol. After 1 year, subjects in the treatment arm had improvement in the FVC of 4.19% (95% confidence interval: -0.57-8.95%), though the difference was not significant.

Taken together, the above studies demonstrate some potential for cyclophosphamide to halt the progression of worsening lung function when administered regularly. A meta-analysis including the above randomized studies, a randomized trial of cyclophosphamide versus azathioprine, and 6 additional prospective, observational studies, also showed a small, statistical improvement in FVC from cyclophosphamide treatment after 1 year, though not in DLCO. (Nannini, West et al. 2008) However, the effects noted in the randomized trials above, and the combined effect in the meta-analysis, are so small as to potentially be clinically insignificant. Additionally, cyclophosphamide did have considerable toxicity in the SSc Lung Study, with increased overall adverse effects especially for mild to moderate leukopenia. (Furst, Tseng et al. 2011) Cyclophosphamide also has been shown in long term follow-up studies to have an increased risk of malignancy and gonadal failure, especially with larger cumulative doses, which can be found with daily therapy. (Manno, Boin 2010)

Ultimately, treatment with cyclophosphamide involves a careful evaluation of the potential benefits and risks for a given patient. Optimal patient selection still needs further research as one larger study identified patients with increased severity of reticular infiltrates on HRCT and greater extent of skin involvement as most likely to benefit from treatment, (Roth, Tseng et al. 2011) while another albeit smaller study showed the opposite. (Yiannopoulos, Pastromas et al. 2007) Since intravenous treatment results in less cumulative dose, which should reduce the potential for side effects, it would seem to be the preferred method of treatment. Additionally, concomitant treatment with low dose steroids would seem prudent, since both randomized trials either directly treated patients with steroids or allowed for simultaneous treatment with low doses of prednisone. A study has found an increased benefit from combining cyclophosphamide with higher doses of steroids, (Pakas, Ioannidis et al. 2002) but this may entail a greater risk of immunosuppression and SSc renal crisis. (Teixeira, Mouthon et al. 2008)

Other Immunosuppressants

Due to the significant toxicity of cyclophosphamide and likely only modest improvements in pulmonary function with treatment of individuals with SSc pulmonary involvement, other potential immunosuppressant agents have been investigated.

Azathioprine

Azathioprine is a purine antagonist that acts as an immunosuppressant by reducing numbers of T, B, and NK cells, and also suppressing autoantibody formation. (Marder, McCune 2007) It is commonly used in organ transplantation and for treatment of autoimmune diseases. In a retrospective review of 11 patients with SSc and deteriorating lung function, the majority of subjects who received 12 months of treatment with azathioprine had improvement in FVC percent predicted. (Dheda, Lalloo et al. 2004) However, when directly compared to oral cyclophosphamide (up to 2 mg/kg daily) in a randomized but unblinded trial including 60 subjects with early diffuse disease, FVC and DLCO percent predicted remained stable at 18 months in the cyclophosphamide group, but decreased significantly in subjects treated with azathioprine(2.5 mg/kg daily). (Nadashkevich, Davis et al. 2006) Ultimately, azathioprine still may have benefit as maintenance therapy after treatment with cyclophosphamide,(Berezne, Ranque et al. 2008, Hoyles, Ellis et al. 2006) or in cases where cyclophosphamide is contraindicated, due to its lower toxicity profile.

Mycophenolate

Mycophenolate mofetil is another immunosuppressant that directly inhibits proliferation of activated lymphocytes and is commonly used in organ transplantation to prevent rejection. (Manno, Boin 2010) Aside from its anti-inflammatory effect, it also may modulate pulmonary TGF-beta expression, which makes it especially appealing in the treatment of fibrotic lung disease. (Guo, Leung et al. 2005) Two small, retrospective studies looked at treating subjects with SSc and ILD on HRCT with mycophenolate and showed that lung function remained stable or improved up to 24 months. (Gerbino, Goss et al. 2008, Zamora, Wolters et al. 2008) A prospective study evaluating twice daily mycophenolate sodium (720 mg BID), a delayed released formulation, found that out of the 14 subjects with findings of SSc and ILD who were treated, 11 had stable or improved lung function after 12 months. A meta-analysis including the above studies as well as 2 additional retrospective studies confirmed that mycophenolate is safe and stabilizes lung function. (Tzouvelekis, Galanopoulos et al. 2012) While all of this is promising, larger, randomized studies are needed prior to using mycophenolate regularly.

Imatinib

Imatinib is an inhibitor of the bcr-abl protein tyrosine kinase used in the treatment of multiple cancers. Like mycophenolate, it has been investigated in the treatment of SSc associated ILD because of its ability to block the TGF-beta pathway, which plays a role in the pathogenesis of fibrosis. (Gordon, Spiera 2011) Aside from case reports and case series, there have been 3 studies attempting to identify its utility. Two of the studies found either an improved FVC percent predicted (Spiera, Gordon et al. 2011) or trend towards an improved FVC percent predicted (Khanna, Saggar et al. 2011) at 12 months.

Both studies however had significant numbers of adverse events, and the third study was stopped prior to completion because of poor tolerability of the medication. (Pope, McBain et al. 2011) At this time, further studies are needed to clarify the role of imatinib in the treatment of ILD associated with SSc, especially with regards to its tolerability.

Rituximab

Since B cells can potentially play a role in promoting fibrogenesis, (Bosello, De Luca et al. 2011) studies have investigated treatment of SSc ILD with rituximab, a monoclonal antibody against CD20, which is a protein found primarily on the surface of B cells. Initial studies in subjects with early SSc disease have shown that the medication leads to reductions in B cell numbers, is well tolerated, and lung function remains stable 6 months after treatment. (Lafyatis, Kissin et al. 2009, Smith, Van Praet et al. 2010) Another study showed continued improvement in FVC and DLCO with 2 years of treatment with rituximab every 6 months. (Daoussis, Liossis et al. 2012) A small, randomized trial adding rituximab to standard treatment regimens already being administered to the patients also showed improvement in the FVC relative to the standard treatment regimen alone group. (Daoussis, Liossis et al. 2012)

As of now, these studies have involved only a small number of subjects and most had early disease. However, there is evidence suggesting that rituximab is well tolerated and could potentially improve lung function, but it still needs further investigation.

Autologous Hematapoietic Stem Cell Transplant

Over the last two decades, several studies have attempted to use autologous stem cell transplantation as a means of treating SSc, the rationale being that it provides a reset for the immune system and therefore decreases and potentially reverses autoimmune damage. (Milanetti, Bucha et al. 2011) Treamtent can either be myeloablative or non-myeloablative. Successful use of stem cell transplantation in a relatively larger number of subjects was first reported by the European Group for Blood and Marrow Transplantation and the European League Against Rheumatism (EBMT/EULAR). (Farge, Passweg et al. 2004) Fifty-seven subjects with refractory severe SSc followed for up to 36 months after autologous stem cell transplantation with conditioning regimens including either a myeloablative or non-myeloablative strategy showed stabilization of vital capacity (VC) and total lung capacity (TLC) over that time. Similar long term results were also seen using only nonmyeloablative conditioning in a combined Dutch and French cohort reported later. (Vonk, Marjanovic et al. 2008) A multicenter study in the US including 34 subjects with a similar disease severity who were followed for up to 8 years after myeloablative autologous stem cell transplantation with high dose immunosuppressive therapy showed stabilization of the DLCO and an increase in the FVC. (Nash, McSweeney et al. 2007)

These positive results have spurred several randomized control trials. One reported recently included 19 subjects who were randomized to either non-myeloablative hematopoietic stem-cell transplantation or intravenous cyclophosphamide administered monthly for 6 months. (Burt, Shah et al. 2011) After 1 year of follow-up, subjects in the transplantation group had increases in mean predicted FVC in comparison to the cyclophosphamide group, which actually decreased over that same span. Additionally, HRCT measurement of lung disease also improved in the transplantation group compared to the cyclophosphamide group. These changes persisted to 24 months. Additionally, several subjects who initially were treated with cyclophosphamide switched into the treatment arm with stem cell transplantation at 1 year. These subjects also saw improvement in FVC, TLC, and extent of disease on HRCT after 1 year. Results from a second trial comparing myeloablative stem cell transplantation to intravenous cyclophosphamide (SCOT) have not been reported.

While all of these results are promising, especially with the randomized data reported more recently, there are still significant risks to treatment with stem cell transplantation. At the current time, it is still not accepted as standard practice. However, with more experience, there may be an opportunity for significant benefits in select patients.

Lung Transplantation

ILD may ultimately not respond to pharmacologic interventions and eventually progress to end stage disease. At this point, lung transplantation, either single of bilateral, is a possible treatment option. Morbidity and mortality associated with the procedure is high, with a large retrospective review showing 1 and 3 year survival rates of 67.6% and 45.9%. (Massad, Powell et al. 2005) However, multiple studies have shown that the risk of transplantation for individuals with SSc is similar to individuals with other conditions, such as idiopathic pulmonary fibrosis, undergoing lung transplantation,(Rosas, Conte et al. 2000, Massad, Powell et al. 2005, Schachna, Medsger et al. 2006, Saggar, Khanna et al. 2010, Shitrit, Amital et al. 2009) and therefore remains a viable option for select individuals.

Pulmonary Arterial Hypertension

The pathogenesis of PAH in SSc is multifactorial, involving a fibrotic, obliterative component, as well as endothelial injury and dysfunction. (Shahane 2013) Basic treatment consists of supportive care and includes oxygen and diuretics. Anticoagulation likely has benefit in individuals with idiopathic PH, but may not be as effective in SSc due to the potential for these individuals to have gastro-intestinal telangectasias and a consequent increased bleeding risk. (Hassoun 2011) High dose calcium channel blockers can be an effective treatment in idiopathic pulmonary arterial hypertension, but only for the small percentage of individuals who have a vasodilator response on acute testing, which is even less common in SSc associated PAH. (Hassoun 2011)

Advanced treatment consists primarily of vasodilatory agents from one of 3 classes of medications: prostaglandins, endothelin receptor antagonists, or phosphodiesterase type 5 inhibitors. More recently, anti-proliferative treatments targeting endothelial and smooth muscle cells have also been investigated. If untreated, increased pulmonary pressures eventually lead to right ventricular failure and death within 2-3 years of the diagnosis being made. (D'Alonzo, Barst et al. 1991) As a result, treatment is generally initiated for patients who are symptomatic (World Health Organization functional class II, III, or IV). Choice of treatment can be complicated and is dependent on disease severity and patient and clinician preferences. Treatment can involve any of the medications below, and most likely will involve a combination of them.

Prostaglandins

Prostacyclin is produced by endothelial cells and acts both as a potent vasodilator through its actions on smooth muscle cells as well as an inhibitor of platelet aggregation through a direct effect on platelets. (Vane, Anggard et al. 1990) When given as a continuous intravenous infusion (i.e. epoprostenol) to individuals with IPAH, it has been shown to decrease pulmonary vascular resistance and mean pulmonary artery pressures greater than standard therapy, and these effects can persist over time with increased dose adjustments. (Rubin, Mendoza et al. 1990, Barst, Rubin et al. 1996, McLaughlin, Genthner et al. 1998) Similar results as well as increased exercise capacity as measured by the 6 minute walk test were seen in an unblinded trial randomizing subjects with SSc to intravenous treatment with epoprostenol versus standard therapy for 12 weeks. (Badesch, Tapson et al. 2000) Increased long term survival relative to historical controls has been seen in cohorts treating IPAH with epoprostenol, (McLaughlin, Shillington et al. 2002, Sitbon, Humbert et al. 2002) and similar results have also been seen when treating individuals with SSc associated PAH. (Badesch, McGoon et al. 2009) The daily management of this treatment can be challenging given the need for a central catheter and pumps to deliver a continuous infusion in patients who may have frequent digital issues resulting in decreased manual dexterity. However, at this time, it is still considered first line therapy for patients with severely incapacitating disease (WHO class IV).

There are 2 additional prostacyclin analogues that are used in the treatment of PAH: treprostinil and iloprost. Treprostinil can be given either subcutaneously, intravenously, or in an inhaled form. In a multi-center, double blind, placebo controlled trial with 470 patients with PAH, subcutaneous treprostinil showed significant differences in symptoms and hemodynamic measurements compared to controls, as well as a small but significant difference in the 6 minute walk distance. (Simonneau, Barst et al. 2002) In the subset of 90 patients who had connective tissue disease, of which half had SSc, similar results were seen,(Oudiz, Schilz et al. 2004) though again the effects were small. Intravenous administration of treprostonil has also been shown to improve dyspnea and 6 minute walk distance. (Tapson, Gomberg-Maitland et al. 2006) Unfortunately, no head to head comparison of epoprostenol and treprostinil exists. Treprostinil may be easier to use than epoprostenol since it does not require refrigeration and subcutaneous administration is likely to be safer than long term intravenous access. However, it still requires significant attention and manipulation since it is administered as a continuous infusion.

Iloprost is much more stable than epoprostenol and can be administered in an aerosolized form. Unfortunately, no studies have been conducted specifically in SSc, or have included large numbers of subjects with SSc. However, there been 3 studies that have shown benefit in subjects with PAH. Two small, uncontrolled studies showed improvement in hemodynamics and 6 minute walk distance at 3 (Olschewski, Ghofrani et al. 2000) and 12 months. (Hoeper, Schwarze et al. 2000) A larger, randomized, placebo-controlled trial also showed decreased dyspnea and an increased 6 minute walk distance after 12 weeks of treatment with inhaled iloprost. (Olschewski, Simonneau et al. 2002) While the inhaled format has shown benefit in the PAH population and provides for easier administration than some of the other possible treatments, the effect of the inhaled dose plateaus after 30-90 minutes, which means that as many as 9 inhalations are needed daily to maintain the clinical effect.

Endothelin Receptor Antagonists

Endothelin-1 is a protein produced by endothelial cells that acts as a very potent vasoconstrictor when binding to endothelin receptor subtype A (ET_A), which is primarily located in smooth muscle cells in the pulmonary vasculature. (Raja, Raja 2011, Rubin 2012) Endothelin-1 can additionally stimulate proliferation of smooth muscle cells (Chua, Krebs et al. 1992) when binding to ET_A receptors as well as endothelin receptor subtype B (ET_B). (Sugawara, Ninomiya et al. 1996, Davie, Haleen et al. 2002) ET_B receptors located on endothelial cells also promote vasodilation. (Hirata, Emori et al. 1993)

Antagonists of endothelin-1 receptors have been developed as treatment for PAH. Currently, two oral medications are still used: bosentan, a non-selective agent, and ambrisentan, a more selective ET_A receptor antagonist. A third ET_A receptor selective agent, sitaxsentan, has been withdrawn from the market due to the potential for fatal hepatotoxicity. Both bosentan and ambrisentan have been shown to be well tolerated, increase exercise capacity and reduce dyspnea after 3-4 months of daily treatment in large, randomized, placebo-controlled trials. (Channick, Simonneau et al. 2001, Rubin, Badesch et al. 2002, Galie, Olschewski et al. 2008) The beneficial effect however seems to be less in SSc associated PAH than in IPAH. An open label, prospective study using daily bosentan in subjects with PAH associated with connective tissue disease, of which the majority had SSc, showed an impressive survival rate of 92% at 48 weeks. (Denton, Hachulla 2011) However, this has not been supported by other retrospective data on bosentan. (Girgis, Mathai et al. 2005) Additionally, a more recent meta-analysis looking at the effect of endothelin receptor antagonists as a class only showed that there is a therapeutic effect, but no confirmed morality benefit. (Ryerson, Nayar et al. 2010).

Phosphodiesterase Type 5 Inhibitors

Nitric oxide (NO) is a potent vasodilator that acts by increasing cyclic guanosine monophosphate (cGMP) levels in smooth muscle cells. (Raja, Raja 2011) Phosphodiesterase type 5 is the main enzyme responsible for degrading cGMP in the lung, (Frumkin 2012) and inhibitors of this enzyme isotype promote continued vasodilation and inhibition of smooth muscle cell growth. (Raja, Danton et al. 2006) Three oral phosphodiesterase type 5 inhibitors are currently used in the treatment of PAH: sildenafil, tadalafil, and vardenafil. A large, randomized, placebo controlled trial of oral sildenafil three times daily for 12 weeks in subjects with PAH showed improvement in exercise capacity by 6 minute walk distance and improved hemodynamics. (Galie, Ghofrani et al. 2005) Doses of 20, 40, and 80 mg of sildenafil were tested, but a significant dose effect was not seen. In a post-hoc, subgroup analysis of the 84 patients in the study with connective tissue disease, about half of whom had SSc and WHO functional class II to III, similar improvements were seen in exercise capacity and hemodynamics irrespective of the dose administered. (Badesch, Hill et al. 2007).

Tadalafil and verdenafil are oral medications dosed once or twice daily, respectively, and have been shown to improve exercise capacity in subjects with PAH in randomized, controlled trials either as monotherapy or in combination with other therapies. (Galie, Brundage et al. 2009, Barst, Oudiz et al. 2011, Oudiz, Brundage et al. 2012, Jing, Jiang et al. 2009, Jing, Yu et al. 2011) In comparison to sildenafil, they also have the benefit of being dosed less frequently daily. However, the studies only included small numbers of individuals with SSc and no analyses of the effect in this particular population has been presented as of yet.

Combination Therapy

In order to attempt to maximize the benefit of medical therapy by targeting different vasodilatory components, multiple studies have focused on combining different treatment classes. Specific combination therapies have included looking at phosphodiesterase inhibitors and endothelin receptor antagonists, endothelin receptor antagonists and a prostaglandin, a phosphodiesterase inhibitor plus a prostaglandin, and a combination of all 3 classes. (Tacket 2013) Many of these studies showed potential benefits, and some have even included subjects with SSc, (Simoneau 2008, Mathai) but none of them have specifically reported the results with respect to the SSc population.

Lung Transplant

Lung transplantation is a viable option when individuals remain symptomatic despite aggressive medical therapy. Although morbidity and mortality from the procedure is significant, individuals with SSc are at similar risk to those with idiopathic PH. (Massad, Powell et al. 2005, Rosas, Conte et al. 2000, Schachna, Medsger et al. 2006, Saggar, Khanna et al. 2010, Shitrit, Amital et al. 2009)

Future Therapies

Over the past decade, much headway has been made in the treatment of PAH, and research is still underway for new therapies. Future possible treatments include new agents in the above classes, as well as tyrosine and ROCK kinase inhibitors, direct cGMP stimulators, vasoactive intestinal peptide analogues, serotonin transport inhibitors, serotonin receptor antagonists, TGF-B inhibitors, nitric oxide synthase, and even gene therapy. (Raja, Raja 2011, Frumkin 2012).

Conclusion

ILD and PAH are the most common causes of mortality in individuals with SSc. Affected individuals typically first present with dyspnea on exertion. Establishing the diagnosis can be difficult, often involving extensive testing, due to the multiple other etiologies of dyspnea in this population. Treatment options for ILD are limited, with cyclophosphamide being the only proven therapy. However, the effects may only be minimal and can involve significant toxicity. Treatment regimens for PAH include vasodilatory agents from different classes of medications and seem to improve patients symptoms and potentially mortality. In both cases, there is still room for improvement, and hopefully new treatments in the future will lead to improved outcomes in this population.

References

Al-Sabbagh, M.R., Steen, V.D., Zee, B.C., Nalesnik, M., Trostle, D.C., Bedetti, C.D. and Medsger, T.A.,Jr, 1989. Pulmonary arterial histology and morphometry in systemic sclerosis: a case-control autopsy study. *The Journal of rheumatology,* 16(8), pp. 1038-1042.

Alton, E. and Turner-Warwick, M., eds, 1988. *Lung Involvement in Scleroderma. In: Systemic Sclerosis (Scleroderma). Black, CM.; Jayson, MIV. (Eds).* Chichester: Wiley.

American Thoracic Society and European Respiratory Society, 2002. American Thoracic Society/European Respiratory Society International Multidisciplinary Consensus Classification of the Idiopathic Interstitial Pneumonias. This joint statement of the American Thoracic Society (ATS), and the European Respiratory Society (ERS) was adopted by the ATS board of directors, June 2001 and by the ERS Executive Committee,

June 2001. *American journal of respiratory and critical care medicine,* 165(2), pp. 277-304.

Badesch, D.B., Hill, N.S., Burgess, G., Rubin, L.J., Barst, R.J., Galie, N., Simonneau, G. and Super Study Group, 2007. Sildenafil for pulmonary arterial hypertension associated with connective tissue disease. *The Journal of rheumatology,* 34(12), pp. 2417-2422.

Badesch, D.B., Mcgoon, M.D., Barst, R.J., Tapson, V.F., Rubin, L.J., Wigley, F.M., Kral, K.M., Raphiou, I.H. and Crater, G.D., 2009. Longterm survival among patients with scleroderma-associated pulmonary arterial hypertension treated with intravenous epoprostenol. *The Journal of rheumatology,* 36(10), pp. 2244-2249.

Badesch, D.B., Tapson, V.F., Mcgoon, M.D., Brundage, B.H., Rubin, L.J., Wigley, F.M., Rich, S., Barst, R.J., Barrett, P.S., Kral, K.M., Jobsis, M.M., Loyd, J.E., Murali, S., Frost, A., Girgis, R., Bourge, R.C., Ralph, D.D., Elliott, C.G., Hill, N.S., Langleben, D., Schilz, R.J., Mclaughlin, V.V., Robbins, I.M., Groves, B.M., Shapiro, S. and Medsger, T.A.,Jr, 2000. Continuous intravenous epoprostenol for pulmonary hypertension due to the scleroderma spectrum of disease. A randomized, controlled trial. *Annals of Internal Medicine,* 132(6), pp. 425-434.

Barst, R.J., Oudiz, R.J., Beardsworth, A., Brundage, B.H., Simonneau, G., Ghofrani, H.A., Sundin, D.P., Galie, N. and Pulmonary Arterial Hypertension and Response to Tadalafil (Phirst) Study Group, 2011. Tadalafil monotherapy and as add-on to background bosentan in patients with pulmonary arterial hypertension. *The Journal of heart and lung transplantation : the official publication of the International Society for Heart Transplantation,* 30(6), pp. 632-643.

Barst, R.J., Rubin, L.J., Long, W.A., Mcgoon, M.D., Rich, S., Badesch, D.B., Groves, B.M., Tapson, V.F., Bourge, R.C., Brundage, B.H., Koerner, S.K., Langleben, D., Keller, C.A., Murali, S., Uretsky, B.F., Clayton, L.M., Jobsis, M.M., Blackburn, S.D., Shortino, D., Crow, J.W. and Primary Pulmonary Hypertension Study Group, 1996. A comparison of continuous intravenous epoprostenol (prostacyclin) with conventional therapy for primary pulmonary hypertension. *The New England journal of medicine,* 334(5), pp. 296-301.

Behr, J. and Furst, D.E., 2008. Pulmonary function tests. *Rheumatology (Oxford, England),* 47 Suppl 5, pp. v65-7.

Berezne, A., Ranque, B., Valeyre, D., Brauner, M., Allanore, Y., Launay, D., Le Guern, V., Kahn, J.E., Couderc, L.J., Constans, J., Cohen, P., Mahr, A., Pagnoux, C., Hachulla, E., Kahan, A., Cabane, J., Guillevin, L. and

Mouthon, L., 2008. Therapeutic strategy combining intravenous cyclophosphamide followed by oral azathioprine to treat worsening interstitial lung disease associated with systemic sclerosis: a retrospective multicenter open-label study. *The Journal of rheumatology*, 35(6), pp. 1064-1072.

Black, C.M., Silman, A.J., Herrick, A.I., Denton, C.P., Wilson, H., Newman, J., Pompon, L. and Shi-Wen, X., 1999. Interferon-alpha does not improve outcome at one year in patients with diffuse cutaneous scleroderma: results of a randomized, double-blind, placebo-controlled trial. *Arthritis and Rheumatism*, 42(2), pp. 299-305.

Bosello, S., De Luca, G., Tolusso, B., Lama, G., Angelucci, C., Sica, G. and Ferraccioli, G., 2011. B cells in systemic sclerosis: a possible target for therapy. *Autoimmunity reviews*, 10(10), pp. 624-630.

Bouros, D., Wells, A.U., Nicholson, A.G., Colby, T.V., Polychronopoulos, V., Pantelidis, P., Haslam, P.L., Vassilakis, D.A., Black, C.M. and Du Bois, R.M., 2002. Histopathologic subsets of fibrosing alveolitis in patients with systemic sclerosis and their relationship to outcome. *American journal of respiratory and critical care medicine*, 165(12), pp. 1581-1586.

Burt, R.K., Shah, S.J., Dill, K., Grant, T., Gheorghiade, M., Schroeder, J., Craig, R., Hirano, I., Marshall, K., Ruderman, E., Jovanovic, B., Milanetti, F., Jain, S., Boyce, K., Morgan, A., Carr, J. and Barr, W., 2011. Autologous non-myeloablative haemopoietic stem-cell transplantation compared with pulse cyclophosphamide once per month for systemic sclerosis (ASSIST): an open-label, randomised phase 2 trial. *Lancet*, 378(9790), pp. 498-506.

Channick, R.N., Simonneau, G., Sitbon, O., Robbins, I.M., Frost, A., Tapson, V.F., Badesch, D.B., Roux, S., Rainisio, M., Bodin, F. and Rubin, L.J., 2001. Effects of the dual endothelin-receptor antagonist bosentan in patients with pulmonary hypertension: a randomised placebo-controlled study. *Lancet*, 358(9288), pp. 1119-1123.

Chua, B.H., Krebs, C.J., Chua, C.C. and Diglio, C.A., 1992. Endothelin stimulates protein synthesis in smooth muscle cells. *The American Journal of Physiology*, 262(4 Pt 1), pp. E412-6.

Clements, P.J., Furst, D.E., Wong, W.K., Mayes, M., White, B., Wigley, F., Weisman, M.H., Barr, W., Moreland, L.W., Medsger, T.A.,Jr, Steen, V., Martin, R.W., Collier, D., Weinstein, A., Lally, E., Varga, J., Weiner, S., Andrews, B., Abeles, M. and Seibold, J.R., 1999. High-dose versus low-dose D-penicillamine in early diffuse systemic sclerosis: analysis of a two-year, double-blind, randomized, controlled clinical trial. *Arthritis and Rheumatism,* 42(6), pp. 1194-1203.

D'alonzo, G.E., Barst, R.J., Ayres, S.M., Bergofsky, E.H., Brundage, B.H., Detre, K.M., Fishman, A.P., Goldring, R.M., Groves, B.M. and Kernis, J.T., 1991. Survival in patients with primary pulmonary hypertension. Results from a national prospective registry. *Annals of Internal Medicine,* 115(5), pp. 343-349.

Daoussis, D., Liossis, S.N., Tsamandas, A.C., Kalogeropoulou, C., Paliogianni, F., Sirinian, C., Yiannopoulos, G. and Andonopoulos, A.P., 2012. Effect of long-term treatment with rituximab on pulmonary function and skin fibrosis in patients with diffuse systemic sclerosis. *Clinical and experimental rheumatology,* 30(2 Suppl 71), pp. S17-22.

Davie, N., Haleen, S.J., Upton, P.D., Polak, J.M., Yacoub, M.H., Morrell, N.W. and Wharton, J., 2002. ET(A) and ET(B) receptors modulate the proliferation of human pulmonary artery smooth muscle cells. *American journal of respiratory and critical care medicine,* 165(3), pp. 398-405.

De Souza, R.B., Borges, C.T., Capelozzi, V.L., Parra, E.R., Jatene, F.B., Kavakama, J., Kairalla, R.A. and Bonfa, E., 2009. Centrilobular fibrosis: an underrecognized pattern in systemic sclerosis. *Respiration; international review of thoracic diseases,* 77(4), pp. 389-397.

Denton, C.P. and Hachulla, E., 2011. Risk factors associated with pulmonary arterial hypertension in patients with systemic sclerosis and implications for screening. *European respiratory review: an official journal of the European Respiratory Society,* 20(122), pp. 270-276.

Desai, S.R., Veeraraghavan, S., Hansell, D.M., Nikolakopolou, A., Goh, N.S., Nicholson, A.G., Colby, T.V., Denton, C.P., Black, C.M., Du Bois, R.M. and Wells, A.U., 2004. CT features of lung disease in patients with systemic sclerosis: comparison with idiopathic pulmonary fibrosis and nonspecific interstitial pneumonia. *Radiology,* 232(2), pp. 560-567.

Dheda, K., Lalloo, U.G., Cassim, B. and Mody, G.M., 2004. Experience with azathioprine in systemic sclerosis associated with interstitial lung disease. *Clinical rheumatology,* 23(4), pp. 306-309.

Edwards, P.D., Bull, R.K. and Coulden, R., 1998. CT measurement of main pulmonary artery diameter. *The British journal of radiology,* 71(850), pp. 1018-1020.

Farge, D., Passweg, J., Van Laar, J.M., Marjanovic, Z., Besenthal, C., Finke, J., Peter, H.H., Breedveld, F.C., Fibbe, W.E., Black, C., Denton, C., Koetter, I., Locatelli, F., Martini, A., Schattenberg, A.V., Van Den Hoogen, F., Van De Putte, L., Lanza, F., Arnold, R., Bacon, P.A.,

Bingham, S., Ciceri, F., Didier, B., Diez-Martin, J.L., Emery, P., Feremans, W., Hertenstein, B., Hiepe, F., Luosujarvi, R., Leon Lara, A., Marmont, A., Martinez, A.M., Pascual Cascon, H., Bocelli-Tyndall, C., Gluckman, E., Gratwohl, A., Tyndall, A. and Ebmt/Eular Registry, 2004. Autologous stem cell transplantation in the treatment of systemic sclerosis: report from the EBMT/EULAR Registry. *Annals of the Rheumatic Diseases,* 63(8), pp. 974-981.

Ferri, C., Valentini, G., Cozzi, F., Sebastiani, M., Michelassi, C., La Montagna, G., Bullo, A., Cazzato, M., Tirri, E., Storino, F., Giuggioli, D., Cuomo, G., Rosada, M., Bombardieri, S., Todesco, S., Tirri, G. and Systemic Sclerosis Study Group of the Italian Society of Rheumatology (SIR-GSSSC), 2002. Systemic sclerosis: demographic, clinical, and serologic features and survival in 1,012 Italian patients. *Medicine,* 81(2), pp. 139-153.

Fischer, A., Swigris, J.J., Groshong, S.D., Cool, C.D., Sahin, H., Lynch, D.A., Curran-Everett, D., Gillis, J.Z., Meehan, R.T. and Brown, K.K., 2008. Clinically significant interstitial lung disease in limited scleroderma: histopathology, clinical features, and survival. *Chest,* 134(3), pp. 601-605.

Frumkin, L.R., 2012. The pharmacological treatment of pulmonary arterial hypertension. *Pharmacological reviews,* 64(3), pp. 583-620.

Furst, D.E., Tseng, C.H., Clements, P.J., Strange, C., Tashkin, D.P., Roth, M.D., Khanna, D., Li, N., Elashoff, R., Schraufnagel, D.E. and Scleroderma Lung Study, 2011. Adverse events during the Scleroderma Lung Study. *The American Journal of Medicine,* 124(5), pp. 459-467.

Gabrielli, A., Avvedimento, E.V. and Krieg, T., 2009. Scleroderma. *The New England journal of medicine,* 360(19), pp. 1989-2003.

Galie, N., Brundage, B.H., Ghofrani, H.A., Oudiz, R.J., Simonneau, G., Safdar, Z., Shapiro, S., White, R.J., Chan, M., Beardsworth, A., Frumkin, L., Barst, R.J. And Pulmonary Arterial Hypertension and Response to Tadalafil (Phirst) Study Group, 2009. Tadalafil therapy for pulmonary arterial hypertension. *Circulation,* 119(22), pp. 2894-2903.

Galie, N., Ghofrani, H.A., Torbicki, A., Barst, R.J., Rubin, L.J., Badesch, D., Fleming, T., Parpia, T., Burgess, G., Branzi, A., Grimminger, F., Kurzyna, M., Simonneau, G. And Sildenafil Use in Pulmonary Arterial Hypertension (Super) Study Group, 2005. Sildenafil citrate therapy for pulmonary arterial hypertension. *The New England journal of medicine,* 353(20), pp. 2148-2157.

Galie, N., Hoeper, M.M., Humbert, M., Torbicki, A., Vachiery, J.L., Barbera, J.A., Beghetti, M., Corris, P., Gaine, S., Gibbs, J.S., Gomez-Sanchez,

M.A., Jondeau, G., Klepetko, W., Opitz, C., Peacock, A., Rubin, L., Zellweger, M., Simonneau, G. and ESC Committee For Practice Guidelines (CPG), 2009. Guidelines for the diagnosis and treatment of pulmonary hypertension: the Task Force for the Diagnosis and Treatment of Pulmonary Hypertension of the European Society of Cardiology (ESC) and the European Respiratory Society (ERS), endorsed by the International Society of Heart and Lung Transplantation (ISHLT). *European heart journal,* 30(20), pp. 2493-2537.

Galie, N., Olschewski, H., Oudiz, R.J., Torres, F., Frost, A., Ghofrani, H.A., Badesch, D.B., Mcgoon, M.D., Mclaughlin, V.V., Roecker, E.B., Gerber, M.J., Dufton, C., Wiens, B.L., Rubin, L.J. and Ambrisentan In Pulmonary Arterial Hypertension, Randomized, Double-Blind, Placebo-Controlled, Multicenter, Efficacy Studies (ARIES) Group, 2008. Ambrisentan for the treatment of pulmonary arterial hypertension: results of the ambrisentan in pulmonary arterial hypertension, randomized, double-blind, placebo-controlled, multicenter, efficacy (ARIES) study 1 and 2. *Circulation,* 117(23), pp. 3010-3019.

Gerbino, A.J., Goss, C.H. and Molitor, J.A., 2008. Effect of mycophenolate mofetil on pulmonary function in scleroderma-associated interstitial lung disease. *Chest,* 133(2), pp. 455-460.

Girgis, R.E., Mathai, S.C., Krishnan, J.A., Wigley, F.M. and Hassoun, P.M., 2005. Long-term outcome of bosentan treatment in idiopathic pulmonary arterial hypertension and pulmonary arterial hypertension associated with the scleroderma spectrum of diseases. *The Journal of heart and lung transplantation : the official publication of the International Society for Heart Transplantation,* 24(10), pp. 1626-1631.

Goldin, J.G., Lynch, D.A., Strollo, D.C., Suh, R.D., Schraufnagel, D.E., Clements, P.J., Elashoff, R.M., Furst, D.E., Vasunilashorn, S., Mcnitt-Gray, M.F., Brown, M.S., Roth, M.D., Tashkin, D.P. and Scleroderma Lung Study Research Group, 2008. High-resolution CT scan findings in patients with symptomatic scleroderma-related interstitial lung disease. *Chest,* 134(2), pp. 358-367.

Gordon, J. and Spiera, R., 2011. Imatinib and the treatment of fibrosis: recent trials and tribulations. *Current rheumatology reports,* 13(1), pp. 51-58.

Guo, H., Leung, J.C., Chan, L.Y., Lui, S.L., Tsang, A.W. and Lai, K.N., 2005. Modulation of intra-pulmonary TGF-beta expression by mycophenolate mofetil in lupus prone MRL/lpr mice. *Lupus,* 14(8), pp. 583-592.

Hachulla, E., Carpentier, P., Gressin, V., Diot, E., Allanore, Y., Sibilia, J., Launay, D., Mouthon, L., Jego, P., Cabane, J., De Groote, P., Chabrol, A.,

Lazareth, I., Guillevin, L., Clerson, P., Humbert, M. and Itinerair-Sclerodermie Study Investigators, 2009. Risk factors for death and the 3-year survival of patients with systemic sclerosis: the French ItinerAIR-Sclerodermie study. *Rheumatology (Oxford, England)*, 48(3), pp. 304-308.

Haimovici, J.B., Trotman-Dickenson, B., Halpern, E.F., Dec, G.W., Ginns, L.C., Shepard, J.A. and Mcloud, T.C., 1997. Relationship between pulmonary artery diameter at computed tomography and pulmonary artery pressures at right-sided heart catheterization. Massachusetts General Hospital Lung Transplantation Program. *Academic Radiology*, 4(5), pp. 327-334.

Harrison, N.K., Mcanulty, R.J., Haslam, P.L., Black, C.M. and Laurent, G.J., 1990. Evidence for protein oedema, neutrophil influx, and enhanced collagen production in lungs of patients with systemic sclerosis. *Thorax*, 45(8), pp. 606-610.

Hassoun, P.M., 2011. Lung involvement in systemic sclerosis. *Presse medicale (Paris, France : 1983)*, 40(1 Pt 2), pp. e3-e17.

Heron, M., Grutters, J.C., Ten Dam-Molenkamp, K.M., Hijdra, D., Van Heugten-Roeling, A., Claessen, A.M., Ruven, H.J., Van Den Bosch, J.M. and Van Velzen-Blad, H., 2012. Bronchoalveolar lavage cell pattern from healthy human lung. *Clinical and experimental immunology*, 167(3), pp. 523-531.

Hirata, Y., Emori, T., Eguchi, S., Kanno, K., Imai, T., Ohta, K. and Marumo, F., 1993. Endothelin receptor subtype B mediates synthesis of nitric oxide by cultured bovine endothelial cells. *The Journal of clinical investigation*, 91(4), pp. 1367-1373.

Hoeper, M.M., Schwarze, M., Ehlerding, S., Adler-Schuermeyer, A., Spiekerkoetter, E., Niedermeyer, J., Hamm, M. and Fabel, H., 2000. Long-term treatment of primary pulmonary hypertension with aerosolized iloprost, a prostacyclin analogue. *The New England journal of medicine*, 342(25), pp. 1866-1870.

Hoyles, R.K., Ellis, R.W., Wellsbury, J., Lees, B., Newlands, P., Goh, N.S., Roberts, C., Desai, S., Herrick, A.L., Mchugh, N.J., Foley, N.M., Pearson, S.B., Emery, P., Veale, D.J., Denton, C.P., Wells, A.U., Black, C.M. and Du Bois, R.M., 2006. A multicenter, prospective, randomized, double-blind, placebo-controlled trial of corticosteroids and intravenous cyclophosphamide followed by oral azathioprine for the treatment of pulmonary fibrosis in scleroderma. *Arthritis and Rheumatism*, 54(12), pp. 3962-3970.

Jing, Z.C., Jiang, X., Wu, B.X., Xu, X.Q., Wu, Y., Ma, C.R., Wang, Y., Yang, Y.J., Pu, J.L. and Gao, W., 2009. Vardenafil treatment for patients with pulmonary arterial hypertension: a multicentre, open-label study. *Heart (British Cardiac Society),* 95(18), pp. 1531-1536.

Jing, Z.C., Yu, Z.X., Shen, J.Y., Wu, B.X., Xu, K.F., Zhu, X.Y., Pan, L., Zhang, Z.L., Liu, X.Q., Zhang, Y.S., Jiang, X., Galie, N. And Efficacy and Safety of Vardenafil in the Treatment of Pulmonary Arterial Hypertension (Evaluation) Study Group, 2011. Vardenafil in pulmonary arterial hypertension: a randomized, double-blind, placebo-controlled study. *American journal of respiratory and critical care medicine,* 183(12), pp. 1723-1729.

Katsumoto, T.R., Whitfield, M.L. and Connolly, M.K., 2011. The pathogenesis of systemic sclerosis. *Annual review of pathology,* 6, pp. 509-537.

Khanna, D., Clements, P.J., Furst, D.E., Korn, J.H., Ellman, M., Rothfield, N., Wigley, F.M., Moreland, L.W., Silver, R., Kim, Y.H., Steen, V.D., Firestein, G.S., Kavanaugh, A.F., Weisman, M., Mayes, M.D., Collier, D., Csuka, M.E., Simms, R., Merkel, P.A., Medsger, T.A.,Jr, Sanders, M.E., Maranian, P., Seibold, J.R. and Relaxin Investigators And The Scleroderma Clinical Trials Consortium, 2009. Recombinant human relaxin in the treatment of systemic sclerosis with diffuse cutaneous involvement: a randomized, double-blind, placebo-controlled trial. *Arthritis and Rheumatism,* 60(4), pp. 1102-1111.

Khanna, D., Saggar, R., Mayes, M.D., Abtin, F., Clements, P.J., Maranian, P., Assassi, S., Saggar, R., Singh, R.R. and Furst, D.E., 2011. A one-year, phase I/IIa, open-label pilot trial of imatinib mesylate in the treatment of systemic sclerosis-associated active interstitial lung disease. *Arthritis and Rheumatism,* 63(11), pp. 3540-3546.

Kim, D.S., Yoo, B., Lee, J.S., Kim, E.K., Lim, C.M., Lee, S.D., Koh, Y., Kim, W.S., Kim, W.D., Colby, T.V. and Kitiaichi, M., 2002. The major histopathologic pattern of pulmonary fibrosis in scleroderma is nonspecific interstitial pneumonia. *Sarcoidosis, vasculitis, and diffuse lung diseases: official journal of WASOG / World Association of Sarcoidosis and Other Granulomatous Disorders,* 19(2), pp. 121-127.

Kowal-Bielecka, O., Kowal, K., Highland, K.B. and Silver, R.M., 2010. Bronchoalveolar lavage fluid in scleroderma interstitial lung disease: technical aspects and clinical correlations: review of the literature. *Seminars in arthritis and rheumatism,* 40(1), pp. 73-88.

Kuriyama, K., Gamsu, G., Stern, R.G., Cann, C.E., Herfkens, R.J. and Brundage, B.H., 1984. CT-determined pulmonary artery diameters in predicting pulmonary hypertension. *Investigative radiology,* 19(1), pp. 16-22.

Lafyatis, R., Kissin, E., York, M., Farina, G., Viger, K., Fritzler, M.J., Merkel, P.A. and Simms, R.W., 2009. B cell depletion with rituximab in patients with diffuse cutaneous systemic sclerosis. *Arthritis and Rheumatism,* 60(2), pp. 578-583.

Le Pavec, J., Launay, D., Mathai, S.C., Hassoun, P.M. and Humbert, M., 2011. Scleroderma lung disease. *Clinical reviews in allergy and immunology,* 40(2), pp. 104-116.

Macgregor, A.J., Canavan, R., Knight, C., Denton, C.P., Davar, J., Coghlan, J. and Black, C.M., 2001. Pulmonary hypertension in systemic sclerosis: risk factors for progression and consequences for survival. *Rheumatology (Oxford, England),* 40(4), pp. 453-459.

Manno, R. and Boin, F., 2010. Immunotherapy of systemic sclerosis. *Immunotherapy,* 2(6), pp. 863-878.

Marder, W. and Mccune, W.J., 2007. Advances in immunosuppressive therapy. *Seminars in respiratory and critical care medicine,* 28(4), pp. 398-417.

Massad, M.G., Powell, C.R., Kpodonu, J., Tshibaka, C., Hanhan, Z., Snow, N.J. and Geha, A.S., 2005. Outcomes of lung transplantation in patients with scleroderma. *World journal of surgery,* 29(11), pp. 1510-1515.

Mayes, M.D., Lacey, J.V.,Jr, Beebe-Dimmer, J., Gillespie, B.W., Cooper, B., Laing, T.J. and Schottenfeld, D., 2003. Prevalence, incidence, survival, and disease characteristics of systemic sclerosis in a large US population. *Arthritis and Rheumatism,* 48(8), pp. 2246-2255.

Mclaughlin, V.V., Archer, S.L., Badesch, D.B., Barst, R.J., Farber, H.W., Lindner, J.R., Mathier, M.A., Mcgoon, M.D., Park, M.H., Rosenson, R.S., Rubin, L.J., Tapson, V.F., Varga, J., American College Of Cardiology Foundation Task Force On Expert Consensus Documents, American Heart Association, American College Of Chest Physicians, American Thoracic Society, I. and Pulmonary Hypertension Association, 2009. ACCF/AHA 2009 expert consensus document on pulmonary hypertension a report of the American College of Cardiology Foundation Task Force on Expert Consensus Documents and the American Heart Association developed in collaboration with the American College of Chest Physicians; American Thoracic Society, Inc.; and the Pulmonary Hypertension Association. *Journal of the American College of Cardiology,* 53(17), pp. 1573-1619.

Mclaughlin, V.V., Genthner, D.E., Panella, M.M. and Rich, S., 1998. Reduction in pulmonary vascular resistance with long-term epoprostenol (prostacyclin) therapy in primary pulmonary hypertension. *The New England journal of medicine,* 338(5), pp. 273-277.

Mclaughlin, V.V., Shillington, A. and Rich, S., 2002. Survival in primary pulmonary hypertension: the impact of epoprostenol therapy. *Circulation,* 106(12), pp. 1477-1482.

Mcnearney, T.A., Reveille, J.D., Fischbach, M., Friedman, A.W., Lisse, J.R., Goel, N., Tan, F.K., Zhou, X., Ahn, C., Feghali-Bostwick, C.A., Fritzler, M., Arnett, F.C. and Mayes, M.D., 2007. Pulmonary involvement in systemic sclerosis: associations with genetic, serologic, sociodemographic, and behavioral factors. *Arthritis and Rheumatism,* 57(2), pp. 318-326.

Medsger, T.A.,Jr, 2003. Natural history of systemic sclerosis and the assessment of disease activity, severity, functional status, and psychologic well-being. *Rheumatic diseases clinics of North America,* 29(2), pp. 255-73, vi.

Milanetti, F., Bucha, J., Testori, A. and Burt, R.K., 2011. Autologous hematopoietic stem cell transplantation for systemic sclerosis. *Current stem cell research and therapy,* 6(1), pp. 16-28.

Mukerjee, D., St George, D., Coleiro, B., Knight, C., Denton, C.P., Davar, J., Black, C.M. and Coghlan, J.G., 2003. Prevalence and outcome in systemic sclerosis associated pulmonary arterial hypertension: application of a registry approach. *Annals of the Rheumatic Diseases,* 62(11), pp. 1088-1093.

Muller, N.L. and Miller, R.R., 1990. Computed tomography of chronic diffuse infiltrative lung disease. Part 1. *The American Review of Respiratory Disease,* 142(5), pp. 1206-1215.

Muller, N.L., Miller, R.R., Webb, W.R., Evans, K.G. and Ostrow, D.N., 1986. Fibrosing alveolitis: CT-pathologic correlation. *Radiology,* 160(3), pp. 585-588.

Nadashkevich, O., Davis, P., Fritzler, M. and Kovalenko, W., 2006. A randomized unblinded trial of cyclophosphamide versus azathioprine in the treatment of systemic sclerosis. *Clinical rheumatology,* 25(2), pp. 205-212.

Nannini, C., West, C.P., Erwin, P.J. and Matteson, E.L., 2008. Effects of cyclophosphamide on pulmonary function in patients with scleroderma and interstitial lung disease: a systematic review and meta-analysis of randomized controlled trials and observational prospective cohort studies. *Arthritis research and therapy,* 10(5), pp. R124.

Nash, R.A., Mcsweeney, P.A., Crofford, L.J., Abidi, M., Chen, C.S., Godwin, J.D., Gooley, T.A., Holmberg, L., Henstorf, G., Lemaistre, C.F., Mayes, M.D., Mcdonagh, K.T., Mclaughlin, B., Molitor, J.A., Nelson, J.L., Shulman, H., Storb, R., Viganego, F., Wener, M.H., Seibold, J.R., Sullivan, K.M. and Furst, D.E., 2007. High-dose immunosuppressive therapy and autologous hematopoietic cell transplantation for severe systemic sclerosis: long-term follow-up of the US multicenter pilot study. *Blood,* 110(4), pp. 1388-1396.

Nikpour, M., Stevens, W.M., Herrick, A.L. and Proudman, S.M., 2010. Epidemiology of systemic sclerosis. *Best practice and research.Clinical rheumatology,* 24(6), pp. 857-869.

Olschewski, H., Ghofrani, H.A., Schmehl, T., Winkler, J., Wilkens, H., Hoper, M.M., Behr, J., Kleber, F.X. and Seeger, W., 2000. Inhaled iloprost to treat severe pulmonary hypertension. An uncontrolled trial. German PPH Study Group. *Annals of Internal Medicine,* 132(6), pp. 435-443.

Olschewski, H., Simonneau, G., Galie, N., Higenbottam, T., Naeije, R., Rubin, L.J., Nikkho, S., Speich, R., Hoeper, M.M., Behr, J., Winkler, J., Sitbon, O., Popov, W., Ghofrani, H.A., Manes, A., Kiely, D.G., Ewert, R., Meyer, A., Corris, P.A., Delcroix, M., Gomez-Sanchez, M., Siedentop, H., Seeger, W. and Aerosolized Iloprost Randomized Study Group, 2002. Inhaled iloprost for severe pulmonary hypertension. *The New England journal of medicine,* 347(5), pp. 322-329.

Ostojic, P. and Damjanov, N., 2006. Different clinical features in patients with limited and diffuse cutaneous systemic sclerosis. *Clinical rheumatology,* 25(4), pp. 453-457.

Oudiz, R.J., Brundage, B.H., Galie, N., Ghofrani, H.A., Simonneau, G., Botros, F.T., Chan, M., Beardsworth, A., Barst, R.J. and Phirst Study Group, 2012. Tadalafil for the treatment of pulmonary arterial hypertension: a double-blind 52-week uncontrolled extension study. *Journal of the American College of Cardiology,* 60(8), pp. 768-774.

Oudiz, R.J., Schilz, R.J., Barst, R.J., Galie, N., Rich, S., Rubin, L.J., Simonneau, G. and Treprostinil Study Group, 2004. Treprostinil, a prostacyclin analogue, in pulmonary arterial hypertension associated with connective tissue disease. *Chest,* 126(2), pp. 420-427.

Pakas, I., Ioannidis, J.P., Malagari, K., Skopouli, F.N., Moutsopoulos, H.M. and Vlachoyiannopoulos, P.G., 2002. Cyclophosphamide with low or high dose prednisolone for systemic sclerosis lung disease. *The Journal of rheumatology,* 29(2), pp. 298-304.

Pandey, A.K., Wilcox, P., Mayo, J.R., Sin, D., Moss, R., Ellis, J., Brown, J. and Leipsic, J., 2010. Predictors of pulmonary hypertension on high-resolution computed tomography of the chest in systemic sclerosis: a retrospective analysis. *Canadian Association of Radiologists journal = Journal l'Association canadienne des radiologistes,* 61(5), pp. 291-296.

Pignone, A., Matucci-Cerinic, M., Lombardi, A., Fedi, R., Fargnoli, R., De Dominicis, R. and Cagnoni, M., 1992. High resolution computed tomography in systemic sclerosis. Real diagnostic utilities in the assessment of pulmonary involvement and comparison with other modalities of lung investigation. *Clinical rheumatology,* 11(4), pp. 465-472.

Pope, J., Mcbain, D., Petrlich, L., Watson, S., Vanderhoek, L., De Leon, F., Seney, S. and Summers, K., 2011. Imatinib in active diffuse cutaneous systemic sclerosis: Results of a six-month, randomized, double-blind, placebo-controlled, proof-of-concept pilot study at a single center. *Arthritis and Rheumatism,* 63(11), pp. 3547-3551.

Pope, J.E., Bellamy, N., Seibold, J.R., Baron, M., Ellman, M., Carette, S., Smith, C.D., Chalmers, I.M., Hong, P., O'hanlon, D., Kaminska, E., Markland, J., Sibley, J., Catoggio, L. and Furst, D.E., 2001. A randomized, controlled trial of methotrexate versus placebo in early diffuse scleroderma. *Arthritis and Rheumatism,* 44(6), pp. 1351-1358.

Raja, S.G., Danton, M.D., Macarthur, K.J. and Pollock, J.C., 2006. Treatment of pulmonary arterial hypertension with sildenafil: from pathophysiology to clinical evidence. *Journal of cardiothoracic and vascular anesthesia,* 20(5), pp. 722-735.

Raja, S.G. and Raja, S.M., 2011. Treating pulmonary arterial hypertension: current treatments and future prospects. *Therapeutic advances in chronic disease,* 2(6), pp. 359-370.

Rosas, V., Conte, J.V., Yang, S.C., Gaine, S.P., Borja, M., Wigley, F.M., White, B. and Orens, J.B., 2000. Lung transplantation and systemic sclerosis. *Annals of Transplantation : Quarterly of the Polish Transplantation Society,* 5(3), pp. 38-43.

Roth, M.D., Tseng, C.H., Clements, P.J., Furst, D.E., Tashkin, D.P., Goldin, J.G., Khanna, D., Kleerup, E.C., Li, N., Elashoff, D., Elashoff, R.M. and Scleroderma Lung Study Research Group, 2011. Predicting treatment outcomes and responder subsets in scleroderma-related interstitial lung disease. *Arthritis and Rheumatism,* 63(9), pp. 2797-2808.

Rubin, L.J., 2012. Endothelin receptor antagonists for the treatment of pulmonary artery hypertension. *Life Sciences,* 91(13-14), pp. 517-521.

Rubin, L.J., Badesch, D.B., Barst, R.J., Galie, N., Black, C.M., Keogh, A., Pulido, T., Frost, A., Roux, S., Leconte, I., Landzberg, M. and Simonneau, G., 2002. Bosentan therapy for pulmonary arterial hypertension. *The New England journal of medicine,* 346(12), pp. 896-903.

Rubin, L.J., Mendoza, J., Hood, M., Mcgoon, M., Barst, R., Williams, W.B., Diehl, J.H., Crow, J. and Long, W., 1990. Treatment of primary pulmonary hypertension with continuous intravenous prostacyclin (epoprostenol). Results of a randomized trial. *Annals of Internal Medicine,* 112(7), pp. 485-491.

Ryerson, C.J., Nayar, S., Swiston, J.R. and Sin, D.D., 2010. Pharmacotherapy in pulmonary arterial hypertension: a systematic review and meta-analysis. *Respiratory research,* 11, pp. 12-9921-11-12.

Saggar, R., Khanna, D., Furst, D.E., Belperio, J.A., Park, G.S., Weigt, S.S., Kubak, B., Ardehali, A., Derhovanessian, A., Clements, P.J., Shapiro, S., Hunter, C., Gregson, A., Fishbein, M.C., Lynch Iii, J.P., Ross, D.J. and Saggar, R., 2010. Systemic sclerosis and bilateral lung transplantation: a single centre experience. *The European respiratory journal : official journal of the European Society for Clinical Respiratory Physiology,* 36(4), pp. 893-900.

Schachna, L., Medsger, T.A.,Jr, Dauber, J.H., Wigley, F.M., Braunstein, N.A., White, B., Steen, V.D., Conte, J.V., Yang, S.C., Mccurry, K.R., Borja, M.C., Plaskon, D.E., Orens, J.B. and Gelber, A.C., 2006. Lung transplantation in scleroderma compared with idiopathic pulmonary fibrosis and idiopathic pulmonary arterial hypertension. *Arthritis and Rheumatism,* 54(12), pp. 3954-3961.

Schioppo, T., Artusi, C., Ciavarella, T., Ingegnoli, F., Murgo, A., Zeni, S., Chighizola, C. and Meroni, P.L., 2012. N-TproBNP as biomarker in systemic sclerosis. *Clinical reviews in allergy and immunology,* 43(3), pp. 292-301.

Schurawitzki, H., Stiglbauer, R., Graninger, W., Herold, C., Polzleitner, D., Burghuber, O.C. and Tscholakoff, D., 1990. Interstitial lung disease in progressive systemic sclerosis: high-resolution CT versus radiography. *Radiology,* 176(3), pp. 755-759.

Shahane, A., 2013. Pulmonary hypertension in rheumatic diseases: epidemiology and pathogenesis. *Rheumatology international, .*

Shitrit, D., Amital, A., Peled, N., Raviv, Y., Medalion, B., Saute, M. and Kramer, M.R., 2009. Lung transplantation in patients with scleroderma:

case series, review of the literature, and criteria for transplantation. *Clinical transplantation,* 23(2), pp. 178-183.

Silver, R.M., Metcalf, J.F., Stanley, J.H. and Leroy, E.C., 1984. Interstitial lung disease in scleroderma. Analysis by bronchoalveolar lavage. *Arthritis and Rheumatism,* 27(11), pp. 1254-1262.

Silver, R.M., Miller, K.S., Kinsella, M.B., Smith, E.A. and Schabel, S.I., 1990. Evaluation and management of scleroderma lung disease using bronchoalveolar lavage. *The American Journal of Medicine,* 88(5), pp. 470-476.

Simonneau, G., Barst, R.J., Galie, N., Naeije, R., Rich, S., Bourge, R.C., Keogh, A., Oudiz, R., Frost, A., Blackburn, S.D., Crow, J.W., Rubin, L.J. and Treprostinil Study Group, 2002. Continuous subcutaneous infusion of treprostinil, a prostacyclin analogue, in patients with pulmonary arterial hypertension: a double-blind, randomized, placebo-controlled trial. *American journal of respiratory and critical care medicine,* 165(6), pp. 800-804.

Sitbon, O., Humbert, M., Nunes, H., Parent, F., Garcia, G., Herve, P., Rainisio, M. and Simonneau, G., 2002. Long-term intravenous epoprostenol infusion in primary pulmonary hypertension: prognostic factors and survival. *Journal of the American College of Cardiology,* 40(4), pp. 780-788.

Smith, V., Van Praet, J.T., Vandooren, B., Van Der Cruyssen, B., Naeyaert, J.M., Decuman, S., Elewaut, D. and De Keyser, F., 2010. Rituximab in diffuse cutaneous systemic sclerosis: an open-label clinical and histopathological study. *Annals of the Rheumatic Diseases,* 69(1), pp. 193-197.

Spiera, R.F., Gordon, J.K., Mersten, J.N., Magro, C.M., Mehta, M., Wildman, H.F., Kloiber, S., Kirou, K.A., Lyman, S. and Crow, M.K., 2011. Imatinib mesylate (Gleevec) in the treatment of diffuse cutaneous systemic sclerosis: results of a 1-year, phase IIa, single-arm, open-label clinical trial. *Annals of the Rheumatic Diseases,* 70(6), pp. 1003-1009.

Steele, R., Hudson, M., Lo, E., Baron, M. and Canadian Scleroderma Research Group, 2012. Clinical decision rule to predict the presence of interstitial lung disease in systemic sclerosis. *Arthritis care and research,* 64(4), pp. 519-524.

Steen, V.D., Conte, C., Owens, G.R. and Medsger, T.A.,Jr, 1994. Severe restrictive lung disease in systemic sclerosis. *Arthritis and Rheumatism,* 37(9), pp. 1283-1289.

Steen, V.D., Graham, G., Conte, C., Owens, G. and Medsger, T.A.,Jr, 1992. Isolated diffusing capacity reduction in systemic sclerosis. *Arthritis and Rheumatism,* 35(7), pp. 765-770.

Steen, V.D. and Medsger, T.A., 2007. Changes in causes of death in systemic sclerosis, 1972-2002. *Annals of the Rheumatic Diseases,* 66(7), pp. 940-944.

Steen, V.D. and Medsger, T.A.,Jr, 2000. Severe organ involvement in systemic sclerosis with diffuse scleroderma. *Arthritis and Rheumatism,* 43(11), pp. 2437-2444.

Strickland, B. and Strickland, N.H., 1988. The value of high definition, narrow section computed tomography in fibrosing alveolitis. *Clinical radiology,* 39(6), pp. 589-594.

Strollo, D. and Goldin, J., 2010. Imaging lung disease in systemic sclerosis. *Current rheumatology reports,* 12(2), pp. 156-161.

Sugawara, F., Ninomiya, H., Okamoto, Y., Miwa, S., Mazda, O., Katsura, Y. and Masaki, T., 1996. Endothelin-1-induced mitogenic responses of Chinese hamster ovary cells expressing human endothelinA: the role of a wortmannin-sensitive signaling pathway. *Molecular pharmacology,* 49(3), pp. 447-457.

Tapson, V.F., Gomberg-Maitland, M., Mclaughlin, V.V., Benza, R.L., Widlitz, A.C., Krichman, A. and Barst, R.J., 2006. Safety and efficacy of IV treprostinil for pulmonary arterial hypertension: a prospective, multicenter, open-label, 12-week trial. *Chest,* 129(3), pp. 683-688.

Tashkin, D.P., Elashoff, R., Clements, P.J., Goldin, J., Roth, M.D., Furst, D.E., Arriola, E., Silver, R., Strange, C., Bolster, M., Seibold, J.R., Riley, D.J., Hsu, V.M., Varga, J., Schraufnagel, D.E., Theodore, A., Simms, R., Wise, R., Wigley, F., White, B., Steen, V., Read, C., Mayes, M., Parsley, E., Mubarak, K., Connolly, M.K., Golden, J., Olman, M., Fessler, B., Rothfield, N., Metersky, M. and Scleroderma Lung Study Research Group, 2006. Cyclophosphamide versus placebo in scleroderma lung disease. *The New England journal of medicine,* 354(25), pp. 2655-2666.

Tashkin, D.P., Elashoff, R., Clements, P.J., Roth, M.D., Furst, D.E., Silver, R.M., Goldin, J., Arriola, E., Strange, C., Bolster, M.B., Seibold, J.R., Riley, D.J., Hsu, V.M., Varga, J., Schraufnagel, D., Theodore, A., Simms, R., Wise, R., Wigley, F., White, B., Steen, V., Read, C., Mayes, M., Parsley, E., Mubarak, K., Connolly, M.K., Golden, J., Olman, M., Fessler, B., Rothfield, N., Metersky, M., Khanna, D., Li, N., Li, G. and Scleroderma Lung Study Research Group, 2007. Effects of 1-year treatment with cyclophosphamide on outcomes at 2 years in scleroderma lung disease. *American journal of respiratory and critical care medicine,* 176(10), pp. 1026-1034.

Teixeira, L., Mouthon, L., Mahr, A., Berezne, A., Agard, C., Mehrenberger, M., Noel, L.H., Trolliet, P., Frances, C., Cabane, J., Guillevin, L. and Group Francais De Recherche Sur Le Sclerodermie (GFRS), 2008. Mortality and risk factors of scleroderma renal crisis: a French retrospective study of 50 patients. *Annals of the Rheumatic Diseases,* 67(1), pp. 110-116.

Theodore, A.C., Tseng, C.H., Li, N., Elashoff, R.M. and Tashkin, D.P., 2012. Correlation of cough with disease activity and treatment with cyclophosphamide in scleroderma interstitial lung disease: findings from the Scleroderma Lung Study. *Chest,* 142(3), pp. 614-621.

Tzouvelekis, A., Galanopoulos, N., Bouros, E., Kolios, G., Zacharis, G., Ntolios, P., Koulelidis, A., Oikonomou, A. and Bouros, D., 2012. Effect and safety of mycophenolate mofetil or sodium in systemic sclerosis-associated interstitial lung disease: a meta-analysis. *Pulmonary medicine,* 2012, pp. 143637.

Van Den Hoogen, F.H., Boerbooms, A.M., Swaak, A.J., Rasker, J.J., Van Lier, H.J. and Van De Putte, L.B., 1996. Comparison of methotrexate with placebo in the treatment of systemic sclerosis: a 24 week randomized double-blind trial, followed by a 24 week observational trial. *British journal of rheumatology,* 35(4), pp. 364-372.

Vane, J.R., Anggard, E.E. and Botting, R.M., 1990. Regulatory functions of the vascular endothelium. *The New England journal of medicine,* 323(1), pp. 27-36.

Vonk, M.C., Marjanovic, Z., Van Den Hoogen, F.H., Zohar, S., Schattenberg, A.V., Fibbe, W.E., Larghero, J., Gluckman, E., Preijers, F.W., Van Dijk, A.P., Bax, J.J., Roblot, P., Van Riel, P.L., Van Laar, J.M. and Farge, D., 2008. Long-term follow-up results after autologous haematopoietic stem cell transplantation for severe systemic sclerosis. *Annals of the Rheumatic Diseases,* 67(1), pp. 98-104.

Wells, A.U., Hansell, D.M., Rubens, M.B., Cullinan, P., Black, C.M. and Du Bois, R.M., 1993. The predictive value of appearances on thin-section computed tomography in fibrosing alveolitis. *The American Review of Respiratory Disease,* 148(4 Pt 1), pp. 1076-1082.

Wells, A.U., Hansell, D.M., Rubens, M.B., King, A.D., Cramer, D., Black, C.M. and Du Bois, R.M., 1997. Fibrosing alveolitis in systemic sclerosis: indices of lung function in relation to extent of disease on computed tomography. *Arthritis and Rheumatism,* 40(7), pp. 1229-1236.

Wells, A.U., Steen, V. and ValentinI, G., 2009. Pulmonary complications: one of the most challenging complications of systemic sclerosis. *Rheumatology (Oxford, England),* 48 Suppl 3, pp. iii40-4.

Yiannopoulos, G., Pastromas, V., Antonopoulos, I., Katsiberis, G., Kalliolias, G., Liossis, S.N. and Andonopoulos, A.P., 2007. Combination of intravenous pulses of cyclophosphamide and methylprednizolone in patients with systemic sclerosis and interstitial lung disease. *Rheumatology international,* 27(4), pp. 357-361.

York, M. and Farber, H.W., 2011. Pulmonary hypertension: screening and evaluation in scleroderma. *Current opinion in rheumatology,* 23(6), pp. 536-544.

Zamora, A.C., Wolters, P.J., Collard, H.R., Connolly, M.K., Elicker, B.M., Webb, W.R., King, T.E.,Jr and Golden, J.A., 2008. Use of mycophenolate mofetil to treat scleroderma-associated interstitial lung disease. *Respiratory medicine,* 102(1), pp. 150-155.

(DLCO) and 6-minute walk (6MWT) test with measurement of oxygen saturation are essential at the time of diagnosis of SSc. Generally, a lung biopsy is not needed in patients with SSc-ILD, except in the case of a discrepancy between clinical manifestations and HRCT findings. Treatment of ILD remains disappointing although many promising therapies are emerging. Cyclophosphamide (CYC), which has been used for 20 years, has recently been evaluated in two prospective randomized studies that failed to demonstrate a major benefit for lung function. Mycophenolate mofetil, azathioprine and rituximab are as alternatives to CYC. Promising cellular and molecular targeted anti-fibrotic therapeutic options have emerged. Lung transplantation can be proposed in the absence of other major organ involvement.

Introduction

SSc is a multisystemic fibrotic disease that affects the skin and internal organs [1]. The prevalence of SSc varies between 200 and 260 cases per million inhabitants in the United States and Australia, 20 and 50 per million in Asia and 100 and 200 per million in Europe [2,3]. SSc incidence ranging from 2.3 to 22.8 cases per 1 million persons per year. Women are more frequently affected than are men (3 to 8 women for one man) [4]. The peak frequency of disease is between 45 and 64 years [5].

Scleroderma has been classified into 2 subsets, limited cutaneous SSc (lcSSc) and diffuse cutaneous SSc (dcSSc), based on clinical and laboratory features [6]. In lcSSc, fibrosis is mainly restricted to the fingers and/or distal limbs and face. Raynaud's phenomenon (RP), the manifestation of vascular disease and marker of tissue ischemia, is present for several years before fibrosis appears. Isolated pulmonary hypertension, that leads to secondary progressive right-sided heart failure, is frequent in the late stage of the disease, and anticentromere antibodies (ACA) occur in 50 to 90% of patients. In dcSSc, fibrosis affects a large area of the skin (proximal to the elbows and/or knees and trunk, face) that becomes evident 1-12 months after the onset of other symptoms. The risk of internal organ involvement is strongly linked to extent and progression of skin thickening. ILD, cardiac disease and renal crisis (SRC), accounts for increased morbidity and mortality, occur predominately in dcSSc. In particular, lung involvement is the major cause of death in SSc. DcSSc is frequently associated with the presence of anti-topoisomerase 1 antibodies (anti Scl-70).

In: Scleroderma   ISBN: 978-1-62618-802-0
Editor: Romain De Winter   © 2013 Nova Science Publishers, Inc.

Chapter II

Interstitial Lung Disease in Systemic Sclerosis: Pathophysiology and Therapy

Paola Cipriani, Vasiliki Liakouli,
Francesco Carubbi, Piero Ruscitti,
Paola Di Benedetto and Roberto Giacomelli
Chair and Clinical Unit of Rheumatology, Department of Biotechnological
and Applied Clinical Science, University of L'Aquila, L'Aquila, Italy

Abstract

Systemic sclerosis or scleroderma (SSc) is an autoimmune disease characterized by a widespread microangiopathy, immune system alterations and fibrosis of the skin and internal organs. Lung involvement is a frequent complication and interstitial lung disease (ILD) represents a leading cause of morbidity and mortality in SSc patients. Unlike idiopathic ILD, SSc-ILD corresponds to non-specific interstitial pneumonia (NSIP) in most cases, whereas usual interstitial pneumonia (UIP) is less frequently encountered. Therefore, the prognosis of SSc-ILD is better than that for idiopathic ILD. However, in a small number of cases, it may progress rapidly to end-stage respiratory insufficiency. Thoracic high-resolution computed tomography (HRCT), pulmonary function tests (PFT) including carbon monoxide diffusing capacity

Visceral involvement can also occur in the absence of cutaneous involvement (*systemic sclerosis sine scleroderma*) [7].

SSc, whether presenting in the limited or diffuse form or sine scleroderma, is a systemic disease with the potential for multiple organ system involvement including the gastrointestinal, cardiac, renal, and pulmonary systems. Pulmonary involvement is common in the course of SSc, and ILD represents one of the two main causes of death in SSc patients [8] since the introduction of angiotensin-converting enzyme inhibitors for renal crisis. Thus, lung involvement has been the target of several clinical studies estimating safety and efficacy of a significant number of therapeutic agents, including cortico-steroids, immunosuppressive and antifibrotic agents, hematopoietic and stem cell transplantation and lung transplantation.

Classification of ILD

ILD is classified on the basis of histopathological data mainly into UIP, NSIP [9]. Unlike idiopathic ILD, which corresponds in most cases to UIP, SSc-ILD corresponds to NSIP in most cases (76%), whereas UIP is less frequently encountered (11%) [10]. A number of cases exhibit end-stage lung fibrosis, and ILD cannot be classified. SSc-ILD has relatively better prognosis than does idiopathic ILD.

NSIP consists in lesions that are homogeneous, at the same stage of evolution, with predominant inflammatory infiltrates, without much destruction or fibrotic lesions while UIP corresponds to heterogeneous lesions at different stages of evolution with foci of young fibroblastic tissue. [10,11]. It is now accepted that lung biopsy is not needed in patients with SSc-ILD, except in the case of a discrepancy between clinical manifestations and HRCT findings. However, outcome is linked more strongly to disease severity at presentation and serial DLCO trends than to histopathologic findings.

Pathophysiology

The underlying mechanism of the pulmonary fibrosis is not completely understood but a complex interplay of vascular injury, inflammation and fibrosis was recently reviewed. Microvascular injury and damage to the endothelial cells appear to be the initiating factors [12]. The increased production of extra-cellular matrix (ECM) proteins by fibroblasts results from abnormal interactions between endothelial cells, mononuclear cells (lymphocytes and monocytes) and fibroblasts, thus leading to the production of fibrosis-inducing cytokines, in a setting of vascular hyperreactivity and tissue hypoxia [13].

Recent animal and human data also suggests that injury to epithelial cells may also play an important role in the pathogenesis [14].

The immune system plays an important role showed by the increased levels of inflammatory and profibrotic cytokines. Either inflammation or initial vascular damage leads to the local production of profibrotic factors such as thrombin and endothelin-1 (ET-1). Thrombin promotes coagulation through the activation of fibrin and promotes the differentiation of fibroblasts into the more metabolically active myofibroblasts [15]. ET-1 is typically considered a local vasoconstrictor but also exerts pro-fibrotic activity by modulating matrix turnover and interacting with transforming growth factor-ß signaling (TGFβ) [16]. ET-1 has been shown to play an important role in ILD based on the elevated ET-1 levels in the plasma and bronchoalveolar lavage fluids (BAL) of patients with ILD [17]. Furthermore, application of bosentan, an endothelin receptor antagonist, in bleomycin rats resulted in significantly higher exercise capacity as a result of improvements in pulmonary hypertension and pulmonary fibrosis [18]. ET-1 and TGFβ and other stimuli can induce connective tissue growth factor production (CTGF), a cytokine that stimulates fibroblast growth factor and up-regulates production of collagen and fibronectin [19]. In lung biopsies of SSc patients, TGFβ expression is increased in the fibrotic lung tissue [20].

B lymphocytes are also early activated in the course of the disease and, by producing autoantibodies, cause fibroblasts to adopt a profibrotic phenotype [21]. Moreover, oxidative stress might play an important role in the pathogenesis of SSc.

Skin fibroblasts, from patients with SSc, spontaneously produce more reactive oxygen species (ROS) than do fibroblasts from healthy controls, depending on the activation of NADPH oxidase (nicotinamide adenine dinucleotide phosphate-oxidase). The inhibition of ROS production by N-acetyl cysteine (NAC) leads to cellular deactivation and decreased collagen production [22].

Clinical Presentation and Diagnosis

The development of ILD in patients with SSc may be slow and progressive. SSc-ILD is often asymptomatic, and clinical manifestations occur at the late stages of the disease. Patients with SSc-ILD may present dry cough, dyspnea on exertion without chest pain and/or general weakness. These symptoms are often ignored by the patient or are masked by joint and/or muscular limitation on exercise. Physical examination reveals "Velcro-like" crackles at the lung bases in the absence of heart failure. At the later stages of ILD, cyanosis and signs of right heart failure may be detected. ILD occurs more commonly in dcSSc. In dcSSc, ILD develops earlier, often in a more severe form at the onset. The prevalence of SSc-ILD may vary from 16% to 100% [23-26]. However, SSc- ILD is detected in approximately 75% out of patients when systematically investigated. About 50% of patients with ILD show an early worsening of PFT (during the first 3 years), even if they are asymptomatic [24, 25], but severe restrictive lung disease (forced vital capacity [FVC] <55%) develops in only a small percentage, lesser than 15%, of these patients [23].

The most sensitive method for detecting early lung disease in scleroderma is to perform PFT. Mild changes in function can be detected before any symptoms develop or changes in chest radiography. However, early ILD cannot be excluded by normal PFT. The most common changes of PFT are either a reduced DLCO or a reduction in lung volumes (FVC) typical of a restrictive ventilator defect with associated reduction in gas exchange [27]. A HRCT scan of the chest is a very sensitive technique for detecting changes in the lung parenchyma. HRCT changes suggestive of ILD include ill-defined, subpleural infiltrates or densities in the posterior segments of the lower lobes, interstitial reticular infiltrates and subpleural honeycombing changes. Both traction bronchiectasis and large cystic changes develop with progressive restricted lung disease. The extent of pulmonary fibrosis, as assessed on HRCT is negatively correlated with FVC and is a powerful predictor of survival [28]. Since SSc-ILD is predominantly subpleural, histological changes are more likely to be found in peripheral lung biopsy compared to other lung locations. Histological findings correlate relatively well with HRCT findings [29]. However, it is now accepted that patients with SSc-ILD, do need lung biopsies, except in the case of a discrepancy between clinical mani-festations and HRCT findings [10].

Bronco-alveolar lavage (BAL) is used to detect inflammation and active alveolitis. Its prognostic value is of unclear value. Although lung biopsies and BAL have provided insight into the pathogenesis and cellular mechanisms of SSc-ILD, they are invasive procedures and are therefore not routinely performed. Furthermore, BAL did not show any predictive value for evaluating the rate of response to CYC in the Scleroderma Lung Study (SLS) [30]. Only, one retrospective study suggests that increased eosinophils in the BAL fluid is associated with a poor prognosis [10]. However, the diagnosis of SSc-ILD is frequently suggested by the constellation of symptoms, physical findings, pulmonary function and HRCT abnormalities.

Prognosis

The prognosis of SSc-ILD is better than the prognosis observed in IPF [25]. The two main features in defining the prognosis of SSc-ILD are immediate, severe ILD based on clinical criteria (dyspnea, crackles), respiratory function (DLCO and/or FVC <70%) and HRCT (extensive lesions with predominant ground glass) and rapidly progressive ILD (defined by a loss of 10% of FVC or 15% of DLCO) during the previous 12 months [31]. Risk factors for serious restrictive lung disease are African-American or Afro-Caribeans races and antitopoisomerase antibodies [32]. Histopathologic distinction between cellular and fibrotic NSIP had no prognostic significance [10]. The survival rate in patients with SSc-ILD, at 5 years is more than 90%; in 1994, it was estimated to be 85% [25]. As far as dcSSc is concerned, the survival at 9 years with ILD was measured at 38% [33]. Severe chronic respiratory insufficiency develops in 16% of patients with SSc-ILD overall [31].

Treatment Corticosteroids

Corticosteroids are used in SSc-ILD for their anti-inflammatory and immunosuppressive properties. Corticosteroids also have anti-fibrosing effects by reducing the synthesis of mucopolysaccharides that are necessary for collagen synthesis [33]. Intravenous infusion of dexamethasone, was shown to improved the vital capacity and post-treatment histopathologic regression was also seen [34]. However, to date, the efficacy of corticosteroids has not been documented in SSc-ILD.

Moreover, a number of studies reported an increased risk of SRC in patients receiving high-dose corticosteroids [35-36]. Thus, low dose corticosteroids (<15 mg/day) are recommended only for patients with severe/worsening ILD [37]. Finally, studies have outlined the therapeutic effects of using a combination of intravenous pulses of cyclophosphamide and methylprednisolone in patients with SSc-ILD [38].

Immunosuppressive Drugs
Cyclophosphamide (CYC)

Cyclophosphamide (CYC), an alkylating agent with immunomodulatory effects, has been used for more than 20 years for SSc-ILD. Its suppressive effects on lymphokine production and lymphocyte function renders it a powerful immunosuppressant [39].

In 1993, a study reported that in 14 patients with SSc-ILD treated with oral CYC (1-2 mg/kg/day) and low dose prednisone (< 10 mg/day) there was a significant improvement in FVC after 6 months compared to entry values. Improvement was maintained at 12 months and 18-24 months and in 12 cases followed for 18-24 months, FVC was stable or improved [40]. Later in 2000, another study analysed 103 patients with scleroderma, 69 had alveolitis and 34 did not. Thirty-nine of the patients with alveolitis were treated with CYC. Lung function outcomes (FVC and DLCO) and survival were improved in patients with alveolitis who received CYC than untreated patients [41].

The association of CYC and corticosteroids was also evaluated in uncontrolled studies and it seems to result in further improvement in lung function tests of SSc patients [42, 43] in spite of the risk of renal crisis. A study revealed that high doses of corticosteroids and CYC had a clinical and radiological beneficial effect after 1 year of treatment. A significant increase in DLCO in 12 months was also reported with this association, but with low dose of prednisone [43].

In contrast, an open study with 14 SSc patients demonstrated only a stabilization of lung parameters during the initial 6 months and deterioration thereafter [44].

In a double-blind multicenter trial (Scleroderma Lung Study) 158 patients with early SSc-ILD, dyspnea, and evidence of active alveolitis were enrolled and randomly assigned to receiving oral CYC (≤2 mg/kg) or placebo daily for one year. Oral daily CYC showed modest clinical efficacy (a small but significant difference in FVC% between treated patients *vs* those receiving placebo) which raised optimism but prompted cautionary advice regarding the use of this toxic drug for these patients.

In particular, the SLS showed that CYC was associated with reduced loss of lung function (FVC and TLC), when compared to the placebo group at the end of the one-year treatment period. The effect of FVC% and TLC% was durable for an additional 6 month after CYC discontinuation but it disappeared after 24 month, although improvement in respiratory symptoms and skin changes persisted. No difference was found for DLCO. Unfortunately, at 2 years, the overall differences between groups were small, especially for PFT, and no significant beneficial effect could be demonstrated [45].

Furthermore, a second prospective trial, the Fibrosing Alveolitis in Scleroderma Trial (FAST), comparing monthly infusion of CYC combined with prednisolone (20 mg on alternate days) followed by azathioprine (AZA) (23 patients) versus placebo (22 patients), showed only a not significant trend toward improvement in FVC (primary outcome) in the treated group. Moreover, no significant improvement in both DLCO values and dyspnea index was observed. These data suggest that treatment of pulmonary fibrosis in SSc with low-dose prednisolone and intravenous CYC followed by AZA stabilizes lung function in a subset of patients with the disease [46].

The main pitfall in these studies concerns the patient's selection. In fact, none of the patients included in studies was selected on the basis of ILD progression, with the exception of the Silver et al. study, in 1993, in which 9 of 14 patients showed a significant decrease in FVC in the 3 to 24 months before study entry [47]. This important lack of data in patients with worsening ILD might partially explain the difficulties to obtain a clinically relevant benefit of CYC in patients with SSc-ILD. Thus, further studies are needed to evaluate whether CYC therapy might be beneficial for patients with worsening ILD.

Azathioprine

Azathioprine (AZA) has also been used for the treatment of SSc-ILD. In 1979, a study based on 19 patients with progressive systemic sclerosis, an AZA long-term therapy, seemed to show, in most cases, to hold the progression of SSc [48]. In particular, in 16 patients, no further deterioration in the lung and kidney manifestations were found. In a randomized non blinded study comparing CYC and AZA, in addition to low dose corticosteroids, FVC and DLCO seemed to remain stable in the CYC group while these values declined in the AZA group [49]. Finally, in a retrospective series of 20 patients with SSc-ILD, intravenous CYC followed by oral therapy with AZA, for worsening ILD, was well tolerated and was associated with stable or improved PFT in 70% and 51.8% of SSc patients at 6 months and 2 years, respectively [50]. Further studies are needed to evaluate whether AZA treatment might be beneficial for patients with SSc-ILD.

Mycophenolate Mofetil

Mycophenolate mofetil (MMF), an inhibitor of lymphocyte proliferation used to control organ transplant rejection, has been tested in several uncontrolled clinical studies and retrospective analyses in SSc-ILD and appears to favorable affect ILD [51-56]. In a large retrospective analysis, 109 patients with or without ILD, were treated with MMF and 63 control subjects receiving other immunosuppressive drugs. Of all patients, experienced adverse reactions with gastrointestinal (GI) tract disturbances and infections. MMF discontinuation was related to disease stabilization in 9%, side effects in 8% and no effect on the disease activity in 14% out of the patients. The Authors reported a significantly lower frequency of clinically significant pulmonary fibrosis in the MMF-treated cohort and significantly better survival rate at 5-yr. No difference between the two groups in terms of modified Rodnan skin score (mRSS) and FVC change was observed [56]. On these basis, is still ongoing in the USA the SLSII (NCT00883129), to evaluate the efficacy and safety of MMF in comparison with oral CYC in 150 patients with SSc-ILD.

Methotrexate

The efficacy of Methotrexate (MTX), a competitive antagonist of folic acid reductase, was also investigated in the treatment of SSc. In a multicenter, randomized double-blind trial, followed by an observational trial of 24 weeks duration, oral MTX has been examined and twenty-nine SSc patients, were allocated to receive weekly injections of either 15 mg MTX or placebo. A favorable response was defined as an improvement of total skin score (TSS) by ≥30%, DLCO by ≥15%, or of the score on a visual analogue scale of general well-being (VAS) by ≥30%, provided that such improvements were not accompanied by persistent digital ulcerations or worsening of DLCO ≥15% [58]. Although the number of patients enrolled in this study were small, these results suggest, that in a group of patients with active systemic sclerosis, low-dose MTX seems to be more effective than placebo according to pre-defined response criteria.

Furthermore, in a multicenter, randomized, placebo-controlled, double-blind trial that was undertaken to evaluate the efficacy of MTX to improve the skin and other disease parameters in early diffuse SSc, 35 patients were treated with MTX and 36 patients received placebo. Treatment was administered for 12 months. The primary outcome measures were skin score (as determined with 2 different indices) and physician global assessment. At study completion, MTX appeared to have a favorable effect on skin scores (mRSS - 4.3 in the MTX group versus 1.8 in the placebo group [$P < 0.009$]). The DLCO was better preserved in the MTX group, although the difference was not significant. Although results of this trial demonstrated a trend in favor of MTX versus placebo in the treatment of early diffuse SSc, the differences between the groups were small and the power to rule out false-negative results was only 50%. These findings do not provide evidence that MTX is significantly effective in the treatment of SSc-ILD [57].

Bosentan

Bosentan, a non-selective endothelin-receptor antagonist, failed to show a beneficial effect in a prospective randomized trial BUILD 2 (Bosentan in Interstitial Lung Disease in Systemic Sclerosis 2) of SSc-ILD. 163 patients with SSc and significant ILD were recruited to this study. The primary efficacy end point was a change in the 6-minute walk distance (6MWD) from baseline up to month 12. Secondary end points included time to death or worsening results of PFTs. The safety and tolerability of bosentan were also assessed. Among the 163 patients, 77 were randomized to receive bosentan, and 86 were randomized to receive placebo. No significant difference between treatment groups was observed for change in the 6MWD up to month 12. No deaths occurred in this study group. Forced vital capacity and diffusing capacity for carbon monoxide remained stable in the majority of patients in both groups. Significant worsening of PFT results occurred in 25.6% of patients receiving placebo and 22.5% of those receiving bosentan. No improvement in exercise capacity was observed in the bosentan-treated group compared with the placebo group, and no significant treatment effect was observed for the other end points. Although many outcome variables were stable, bosentan did not reduce the frequency of clinically important worsening. These data do not support the use of endothelin receptor antagonists as therapy for ILD secondary to SSc [59]. Six minute walk test was found to be reproducible in the short term but lacked construct validity with PFT and exhibited poor reproducibility at a time interval of one year [60]. Furthermore, bosentan treatment in patients with IPF did not show superiority over placebo on 6MWD up to month 12. A trend in delayed time to death or disease progression, and improvement in QOL, was observed with bosentan [61]. To demonstrate that bosentan delays IPF worsening or death, a randomized, controlled trial (BUILD3) was designed. The primary endpoint was time to IPF worsening (a confirmed decrease from baseline in FVC $\geq 10\%$ and diffusing capacity of the lung for carbon monoxide $\geq$ 15%, or acute exacerbation of IPF) or death up to end of study. Effects of bosentan on health-related quality of life, dyspnea, and the safety and tolerability of bosentan were also investigated. The primary objective in the Bosentan Use in Interstitial Lung Disease-3 trial was not met and the safety profile for bosentan was similar to that observed in other trials [62].

Tyrosine Kinase Inhibitors

Transforming growth factor β (TGFβ) and platelet-derived growth factor (PDGF) play a critical role in SSc-ILD pathogenesis and in the last years these 2 molecules were considered therapeutic target to prevent fibrosis. In particular, imatinib, a potent inhibitor of c-abl kinases, prevented TGFβ-induced extracellular matrix gene expression and cell proliferation in a mouse with bleomycin-induced pulmonary fibrosis. In cultured scleroderma fibroblasts, stimulation with TGF-β and PDGF was abrogated by the addition of imatinib [63]. Sporadic cases of CTD interstitial lung disease refractory to standard regimens responded well to imatinib [64,65]. In a preliminary study, 5 patients with advanced SSc-ILD received a combination of intravenous CYC and oral imatinib. Treatment was well tolerated but led to a clinical improvement in only 1 patient with mild ILD [66]. Recently, a phase I/IIa open-label pilot study of imatinib in patients with SSc-related active ILD, was performed to assess the safety and efficacy of imatinib. In this study, were recruited 20 SSc patients with FVC of <85% predicted, dyspnea on exertion, and presence of a ground-glass appearance on HRCT. Patients received oral therapy with imatinib (up to 600 mg/day) for a period of 1 year. Adverse events were recorded, pulmonary function was tested, and the mRSS was assessed every 3 months. The course of changes in lung function, the Health Assessment Questionnaire (HAQ) disability index (DI), and the mRSS were modeled over the period of study to explore treatment efficacy. Of the 20 SSc patients, 12 completed the study, 7 discontinued because of adverse events (AEs), and 1 patient was lost to follow-up. Treatment with imatinib showed a trend toward improvement in the FVC% and a significant improvement in mRSS. Use of high-dose daily therapy with imatinib (600 mg/day) in SSc patients with ILD was associated with a large number of AEs. AEs suggests that dosages of imatinib lower than 600 mg/day may be appropriate and that further dose ranging analysis is needed in order to understand the therapeutic index of imatinib in SSc [67]. Dasatinib, a tyrosine kinase inhibitor with targets similar to imatinib, was reported to potently inhibit the synthesis of extracellular matrix *in vitro* and *in vivo* at biologically relevant concentrations [68]. An open label study was performed to evaluate the safety of dasatinib in the treatment of scleroderma pulmonary interstitial fibrosis" (Clinical Trial Registration Number: NCT00764309). Thus, might be promising drugs for the treatment of patients with SSc.

Anti-IL-13 Antibody

IL-13, a profibrotic cytokine, is a potent stimulator of fibroblast proliferation and collagen production [69]. IL-13 was found to be increased in SSc patients and to sustained the immunological and fibrotic process [70, 71]. Overexpression of IL-13 in mice causes severe lung fibrosis [72, 73] while IL-13 neutralization, inhibits fibrosis in murine models of bleomycin-induced lung damage [74]. A randomized, double-blinded, placebo controlled, multiple-dose, multi-center pilot study, to assess safety, tolerability, pharmacokinetics and pharmacodynamics of intravenous doses of a QAX576 (a fully human monoclonal antibody against human IL-13) in patients with pulmonary fibrosis secondary to SSc has been completed and results are awaited (Clinical Trial Registration Number: NCT00581997). Finally, an open-label, multi-center study, with a single intravenous dose of QAX576 to determine IL-13 production in patients with IPF has been completed and results are always awaited with interest (NCT00532233).

Anti-IL-6 Antibody

Many reports have suggested that IL-6 is involved in SSc pathogenesis. IL-6 expression is reportedly high in both the skin and serum of SSc patients and its elevation was found to correlate with C-reactive protein (CRP) and extent of skin fibrosis [75]. More recently, was found that serum IL-6 levels appear to be predictive of early disease progression in patients with mild SSc-ILD, and could be used to target treatment in this group, if confirmed by prospective studies [76]. Blocking of IL-6 *in vitro* decreased collagen production, and in the bleomycin model, IL-6 deficiency attenuated lung fibrosis [77]. To examine the effect of blockade of IL-6 on SSc, tocilizumab, an anti-IL-6 soluble receptor monoclonal antibody, was administered in two patients with dcSSc over 6 months. After tocilizumab treatment, both patients showed softening of the skin with reductions of 50.7% and 55.7% in the total z-score of Vesmeter hardness and 51.9% and 23.0% in the mRTSS, respectively. However, the fibrotic changes in the lung in the other patient remained unchanged [78]. To estimate potential effects on skin or lung fibrosis, larger randomised, placebo-controlled, prospective trials are needed.

Rituximab

Recent experimental and clinical evidences in mouse models and in SSc patients suggest a role for B cells in inflammation and fibrosis. Levels of B lymphocytes were found to be elevated in lungs of patients with SSc-ILD [79]. Rituximab is a chimeric monoclonal antibody and its mechanism of action is directed against the CD20 antigen on the surfaces of B lymphocytes. In a SSc mouse model, anti-mouse CD20 monoclonal antibody treatment depleted circulating and tissue B cells and suppressed skin fibrosis in newborn mice [80]. Improvement of SSc-ILD with rituximab was reported in isolated case reports [81,82]. More recently, 14 SSc patients were randomized to receive 4 weekly pulses of rituximab at baseline and at 6 months in addition to standard treatment or standard treatment [83]. In the 8 patients receiving rituximab,

FVC and DLCO significantly increased at 1 year but decreased in the control group. Moreover, skin fibrosis improved significantly in the rituximab group at 1 year. Larger scale, multicenter, RCTs are needed to confirm these possible beneficial effects of Rituximab in SSc.

N-Acetyl Cysteine (NAC)

N-acetyl cysteine (NAC) showed beneficial effects for patients with IPF [84]. Recently, a retrospective study investigated data from SSc patients who underwent therapy with high-dose intravenous NAC at a dosage of 15 mg/Kg/h for 5 consecutive hours every 14 days. The primary endpoint of this study was the change between baseline and month 24 in DLCO. The secondary endpoints were: vital capacity (VC), forced expired volume in 1 sec (FEV1), total lung capacity (TLC), scores of HRCT of the chest, number of adverse effects. After NAC therapy median values of DLCO, VC and TLC were significantly increased. The Authors did not observe any significant changes from baseline in FEV1 value and HRTC score. The improvement in lung function was more evident in SSc patients without radiological signs of pulmonary fibrosis than in patients with pulmonary fibrosis. In SSc patients with mild-moderate pulmonary fibrosis intravenous NAC administration slows the rate of deterioration of DLCO, VC and TLC. Finally, the Authors concluded that long-term therapy with intravenous NAC ameliorates pulmonary function tests in SSc patients [85].

Hematopoietic and Stem Cell Transplantation

Immunoablative therapy followed by autologous hematopoietic stem cell transplantation (HSCT) has been proposed for several years for the treatment of autoimmune disorders refractory to conventional treatments. The rationale for HSCT in autoimmune diseases is the ablation of an aberrant or self-reactive immune system by chemotherapy and regeneration of a new and hopefully self-tolerant immune system from hematopoietic stem cells [86]. The ASSIST (American Scleroderma Stem Cell versus Immune Suppression Trial) an open-label, randomized, controlled phase 2 trial, was launched in 2006 to compare safety and efficacy of autologous non-myeloablative HSCT compared with the standard of care, CYC. Patients were eligible if they were aged younger than 60 years and had diffuse systemic sclerosis with an mRSS of more than 14, and with evidence of lung, heart, or gastrointestinal organ involvement. Patients with restricted skin involvement (mRSS<14) were eligible only if they had coexistent lung involvement. Exclusion criteria were end stage organ failure, extensive pretreatment with CYC (more than 6 previous intravenous injections of CYC), and common reasons that preclude participation in a trial. The primary outcome for all enrolled patients was improvement at 12 months follow–up, defined as a decrease in mRSS (>25% for those with initial mRSS>14) or an increase in FVC by more than 10%. In this study, non-myeloablative HSCT significantly improved FVC, decreased disease lung volume, and showed that SSc-ILD might be at least partially reversed with continued improvement in lung function for at least 2 years after transplantation. If patients undertaken this procedure, in early phases of the disease, with careful precardiac assessment, HSCT has little morbidity and improves lung function, whereas delaying of transplantation through treatment with standard of care (CYC) allows disease progression, increases transplantation risk, and might contraindicate HSCT [87].

A randomized study of rituximab plus rabbit anti-thymocyte globulin (rATG) plus CYC *vs*. rATG plus CYC plus hematopoietic stem cell support in patients with SSc (Autologous Systemic Sclerosis Immune Suppression Trial - II ASSIST-II) is currently in progress by recruiting patients (NCT01445821). The investigators in this study propose that a conditioning regimen incorporating B cell depletion using CD20 monoclonal antibody (rituximab) with high dose CYC and rabbit ATG will improve response rate and duration in patients receiving HSCT, when compared to a conditioning regimen of high dose CYC and rabbit ATG regimen with hematopoietic stem cell support alone. Moreover, cell based therapy can indeed be a treatment choice in future for SSc-ILD. Bone marrow derived stem cells are important in the recovery of the lungs from injury, and that administering bone marrow derived mesenchymal stem cells (MSCs) can accelerate lung repair [88]. In 2008, another study also supported this hypothesis, stating that the MSCs differentiated into alveolar epithelial cells, and the transplanted cells curtailed lung injury and fibrosis [89]. Stem cells have the potential to differentiate into all cell types and are considered a valuable source of cells for transplantation therapies. However, the risk of tumor progression after transplantation remains a critical issue. In order to circumvent this problem, another study was planned showing a different approach to cell-based therapy, and alveolar type II cells were transplanted. The study demonstrated the potential of intra tracheal transplantation of alveolar type II cells to reverse the fibrogenic process in damaged lung tissue, thus becoming a promising therapy for the future treatment of fibrotic lung diseases [90].

Lung Transplantation

Lung transplantation may be considered, in the absence of other visceral involvement, an option for patients with severe SSc-ILD who are not responsive to pharmacologic interventions. Carefully selected SSc patients undergoing lung transplantation have acceptable morbidity and mortality comparable to patients undergoing lung transplantation for IPF, as suggested by recent studies [91-93]. However, in patients with SSc, the number of early deaths was increased but not significantly. Lung transplantation may be considered a viable therapeutic option in patients with end-stage lung dysfunction resulting from SSc.

Conclusion

In SSc, pulmonary involvement is common and ILD represents one of the two main causes of death. However, a gold standard treatment for SSC-ILD is not yet well established. A better understanding of the pathophysiology of the disease, is greatly needed and will allow more effective targeted therapy. Because none of the patients included in retrospective or prospective studies was selected on the basis of progression of ILD, further studies are needed to evaluate whether conventional anti-rheumatic drugs therapy might be beneficial for patients with worsening ILD. Looking forward a better selection of patient subsets, associated with the emerging promising cellular and molecular targeted anti-fibrotic therapeutic options might improve our therapeutic possibilities and prognosis.

References

[1]   Medsger TA. Systemic sclerosis (scleroderma): clinical aspects. In: Koopman WJ, ed. Arthritis and allied conditions: a textbook of rheumatology. Philadelphia: Williams & Wilkins, 1997:1433-65.

[2]   LeRoy EC, Black C, Fleischmajer R, Jablonska S, Krieg T, Medsger TA Jr, Rowell N, Wollheim F. Scleroderma (systemic sclerosis): classification, subsets and pathogenesis. *J. Rheumatol.* 1998 ; 15:202-5

[3]   Ranque B, Mouthon L. Geoepidemiology of systemic sclerosis. *Autoimmun Rev.* 2009 Nov 10.

[4]   Le Guern V, Mahr A, Mouthon L, Jeanneret D, Carzon M, Guillevin L. Prevalence of systemic sclerosis in a French multi-ethnic county. *Rheumatology* (Oxford) 2004;43:1129–37.

[5]   Chifflot H, Fautrel B, Sordet C, Chatelus E, Sibilia J. Incidence and prevalence of systemic sclerosis: a systematic literature review. *Semin Arthritis Rheum.* 2008;37: 223–35.

[6]   Mayes MD, Lacey Jr JV, Beebe-Dimmer J, Gillespie BW, Cooper B, Laing TJ, et al. Prevalence, incidence, survival, and disease characteristics of systemic sclerosis in a large US population. *Arthritis Rheum.* 2003;48:2246–55.

[7]   Poormoghim H, Lucas M, Fertig N, Medsger TA. Systemic sclerosis sine scleroderma: demographic, clinical, and serologic features and survival in forty-eight patients.*Arthritis Rheum.* 2000 Feb;43(2):444-5.

[8]   Steen VD, Medsger TA. Changes in causes of death in systemic sclerosis, 1972–2002. *Ann. Rheum. Dis.* 2007;66:940–4.

[9]   American Thoracic Society/European Respiratory Society International Multidisciplinary Consensus Classification of the Idiopathic Interstitial Pneumonias. This joint statement of the American Thoracic Society (ATS), and the European Respiratory Society (ERS) was adopted by the ATS board of directors, June 2001and by the ERS Executive Committee, June 2001. *Am. J. Respir. Crit. Care Med.* 2002;165:277–304.

[10]   Bouros D, Wells AU, Nicholson AG, Colby TV, Polychronopoulos V, Pantelidis P, et al. Histopathologic subsets of fibrosing alveolitis in patients with systemic sclerosis and their relationship to outcome. *Am. J. Respir. Crit. Care Med.* 2002;165:1581–6.

[11]   Kim EA, Lee KS, Johkoh T, Kim TS, Suh GY, Kwon OJ, et al. Interstitial lung diseases associated with collagen vascular diseases: radiologic and histopathologic findings. *Radiographics* 2002;22:S151–65.

[12]   Beon M, Harley RA, Wessels A, Silver RM, Ludwicka-Bradley A. Myofibroblast induction and microvascular alteration in scleroderma lung fibrosis. *Clin. Exp. Rheumatol.* 2004 Nov-Dec;22(6):733-42.

[13]   Tamby MC, Chanseaud Y, Guillevin L, Mouthon L. New insights into the pathogenesis of systemic sclerosis. *Autoimmun. Rev.* 2003;2:152–7.

[14] Hoyles RK, Khan K, Shiwen X, Howat SL, Lindahl GE, Leoni P, du Bois RM, Wells AU, Black CM, Abraham DJ, Denton CP. Fibroblast-specific perturbation of transforming growth factor beta signaling provides insight into potential pathogenic mechanisms of scleroderma-associated lung fibrosis: exaggerated response to alveolar epithelial injury in a novel mouse model. *Arthritis Rheum.* 2008 Apr;58(4):1175-88. doi: 10.1002/art.23379.

[15] Bogatkevich GS, Gustilo E, Oates JC, Feghali-Bostwick C, Harley RA, Silver RM, Ludwicka-Bradley A. Distinct PKC isoforms mediate cell survival and DNA synthesis in thrombin-induced myofibroblasts. *Am. J. Physiol. Lung Cell Mol. Physiol.* 2005 Jan;288(1):L190-201. Epub 2004 Sep 24.

[16] Shi-Wen X, Chen Y, Denton CP, Eastwood M, Renzoni EA, Bou-Gharios G, Pearson JD, Dashwood M, du Bois RM, Black CM, Leask A, Abraham DJ. Endothelin-1 promotes myofibroblast induction through the ETA receptor via a rac/phosphoinositide 3-kinase/Akt-dependent pathway and is essential for the enhanced contractile phenotype of fibrotic fibroblasts. *Mol. Biol. Cell.* 2004 Jun;15(6):2707-19. Epub 2004 Mar 26.

[17] Odoux C, Crestani B, Lebrun G, Rolland C, Aubin P, Seta N, Kahn MF, Fiet J, Aubier M. Endothelin-1 secretion by alveolar macrophages in systemic sclerosis. *Am. J. Respir. Crit. Care Med.* 1997 Nov;156(5):1429-35.

[18] Schroll S, Arzt M, Sebah D, Nüchterlein M, Blumberg F, Pfeifer M. Improvement of bleomycin-induced pulmonary hypertension and pulmonary fibrosis by the endothelin receptor antagonist Bosentan. *Respir. Physiol. Neurobiol.* 2010 Jan 31;170(1):32-6. doi: 10.1016/j.resp.2009.11.005. Epub 2009 Nov 28.

[19] Krieg T, Abraham D, Lafyatis R. Fibrosis in connective tissue disease: the role of the myofibroblast and fibroblast-epithelial cell interactions. *Arthritis Res. Ther.* 2007;9 Suppl 2:S4. Review.

[20] Corrin B, Butcher D, McAnulty BJ, Dubois RM, Black CM, Laurent GJ, Harrison NK. Immunohistochemical localization of transforming growth factor-beta 1 in the lungs of patients with systemic sclerosis, cryptogenic fibrosing alveolitis and other lung disorders. *Histopathology.* 1994 Feb;24(2):145-50.

[21] Bosello S, De Luca G, Tolusso B, Lama G, Angelucci C, Sica G, Ferraccioli G. B cells in systemic sclerosis: a possible target for therapy.

Autoimmun. Rev. 2011 Aug;10(10):624-30. doi: 10.1016/j.autrev.2011. 04.013. Epub 2011 Apr 22. Review.

[22] Sambo P, Baroni SS, Luchetti M, Paroncini P, Dusi S, Orlandini G, et al. Oxidative stress in scleroderma: maintenance of scleroderma fibroblast phenotype by the constitutive up-regulation of reactive oxygen species generation through the NADPH oxidase complex pathway. *Arthritis Rheum.* 2001;44:2653–64.

[23] Preliminary criteria for the classification of systemic sclerosis (scleroderma). Subcommittee for scleroderma criteria of the American Rheumatism Association Diagnostic and Therapeutic Criteria Committee. *Arthritis Rheum.* 1980;23:581–90.

[24] Steen VD, Medsger Jr TA. Severe organ involvement in systemic sclerosis with diffuse scleroderma. *Arthritis Rheum.* 2000;43:2437–44.

[25] Wells AU, Cullinan P, Hansell DM, Rubens MB, Black CM, Newman-Taylor AJ, et al. Fibrosing alveolitis associated with systemic sclerosis has a better prognosis than lone cryptogenic fibrosing alveolitis. *Am. J. Respir. Crit. Care Med.* 1994;149: 1583–90.

[26] Scussel-Lonzetti L, Joyal F, Raynauld JP, Roussin A, Rich E, Goulet JR, et al. Predicting mortality in systemic sclerosis: analysis of a cohort of 309 French Canadian patients with emphasis on features at diagnosis as predictive factors for survival. *Medicine* (Baltimore) 2002;81:154–67.

[27] Wells AU, Rubens MB, du Bois RM, Hansell DM. Serial CT in fibrosing alveolitis: prognostic significance of the initial pattern. AJR *Am. J. Roentgenol.* 1993; 161:1159–65. [PubMed:8249719]

[28] Nakamura Y, Chida K, Suda T, Hayakawa H, Iwata M, Imokawa S, et al. Nonspecific interstitial pneumonia in collagen vascular diseases: comparison of the clinical characteristics and prognostic significance with usual interstitial pneumonia. *Sarcoidosis Vasc. Diffuse Lung Dis.* 2003; 20:235–41. [PubMed: 14620168]

[29] Wells AU, Hansell DM, Rubens MB, Cullinan P, Black CM, du Bois RM. The predictive value of appearances on thin-section computed tomography in fibrosing alveolitis. *Am. Rev. Respir. Dis.* 1993; 148:1076–82. [PubMed: 8214928]

[30] Tashkin DP, Elashoff R, Clements PJ, Goldin J, Roth MD, Furst DE, Arriola E, Silver R, Strange C, Bolster M, Seibold JR, Riley DJ, Hsu VM, Varga J, Schraufnagel DE, Theodore A, Simms R, Wise R, Wigley F, White B, Steen V, Read C, Mayes M, Parsley E, Mubarak K, Connolly MK, Golden J, Olman M, Fessler B, Rothfield N, Metersky M; Scleroderma Lung Study Research Group. Cyclophosphamide versus

placebo in scleroderma lung disease. *N. Engl. J. Med.* 2006 Jun 22;354(25):2655-66.

[31] Steen VD, Conte C, Owens GR, Medsger TA. Severe restrictive lung disease in systemic sclerosis. *Arthritis Rheum.* 1994;37:1283–9.

[32] Greidinger EL, Flaherty KT, White B, Rosen A, Wigley FM, Wise RA. African-American race and antibodies to topoisomerase I are associated with increased severity of scleroderma lung disease. *Chest.* 1998 Sep;114(3):801-7.

[33] Durant S, Duval D, Homo-Delarche F. Factors involved in the control of fibroblast proliferation by glucocorticoids: a review. *Endocr. Rev.* 1986;7:254–69.

[34] Pai BS, Srinivas CR, Sabitha L, Shenoi SD, Balachandran CN, Acharya S. Efficacy of dexamethasone pulse therapy in progressive systemic sclerosis. *Int. J. Dermatol.* 1995 Oct;34(10):726-8.

[35] Steen VD, Medsger Jr TA. Case–control study of corticosteroids and other drugs that either precipitate or protect from the development of scleroderma renal crisis. *Arthritis Rheum.* 1998;41:1613–9.

[36] DeMarco PJ, Weisman MH, Seibold JR, Furst DE, Wong WK, Hurwitz EL, et al. Predictors and outcomes of scleroderma renal crisis: the high-dose versus lowdose D-penicillamine in early diffuse systemic sclerosis trial. *Arthritis Rheum.* 2002;46:2983–9.

[37] Teixeira L, Mouthon L, Mahr A, Berezne A, Agard C, Mehrenberger M, et al. Mortality and risk factors of scleroderma renal crisis: a French retrospective study of 50 patients. *Ann. Rheum. Dis.* 2008;67:110–6.

[38] Griffiths B, Miles S, Moss H, Robertson R, Veale D, Emery P. Systemic sclerosis and interstitial lung disease: a pilot study using pulse intravenous methylprednisolone and cyclophosphamide to assess the effect on high resolution computed tomography scan and lung function.. *J. Rheumatol.* 2002 Nov;29(11):2371-8.

[39] Rang HP, Dale MM, Ritter JM, Flower R: Cancer chemotherapy. In: Rang & Dale's *Pharmacology. Churchill Livingstone Elsevier* 2008: 724

[40] Silver RM, Warrick JH, Kinsella MB, Staudt LS, Baumann MH, Strange C. Cyclophosphamide and low-dose prednisone therapy in patients with systemic sclerosis (scleroderma) with interstitial lung disease. *J. Rheumatol.* 1993 May;20(5):838-44.

[41] White B, Moore WC, Wigley FM, Xiao HQ, Wise RA. Cyclophosphamide is associated with pulmonary function and survival benefit in patients with scleroderma and alveolitis. *Ann. Intern Med.* 2000;132:947–54.

[42] Pakas I, Ioannidis JPA, Malagari K, Skopouli FN, Moutsopoulos HM, Vlachoyiannopoulos PG et al. (2002). Cyclophosphamide with low or high dose prednisolone for systemic sclerosis lung disease. *J. Rheumatol.* 298-304.

[43] Giacomelli R, Valentini G, Salsano F, Cipriani P, Sambo P, Conforti ML et al. (2002) Cyclophosphamide pulse regimen in the treatment of alveolitis in systemic sclerosis. *J. Rheumatol.* 29:731–736.

[44] Griffithis B, Miles S, Mos H, Robertson R, Veale D, Emery P (2002) Systemic sclerosis and interstitial lung disease: a pilot study using oulse intravenous methylprednisolone and cyclophosphamide to assess the effect on high resolution computed tomography scan and lung function. *J. Rheumatol.* 29:2371–2378.

[45] Tashkin DP, Elashoff R, Clements PJ, Goldin J, Roth MD, Furst D, for the Scleroderma Lung Study Research Group et al. (2006). Cyclophosphamide versus placebo in scleroderma lung disease. *N. Engl. J. Med.* 354:2655–2666.

[46] Hoyles RK, Ellis RW, Wellsbury J, Lees B, Newlands P, Goh NSL et al. (2006) A Multicenter, prospective, randomized, double-blind, placebo-controlles trial os corticosteroids and intravenous cyclophosphamide followed by oral azathioprine for the treatment of pulmonary fibrosis in scleroderma. *Arthritis Rheum.* 54:3692–3970.

[47] Silver RM, Warrick JH, Kinsella MB, Staudt LS, Baumann MH, Strange C. Cyclophosphamide and low-dose prednisone therapy in patients with systemic sclerosis (scleroderma) with interstitial lung disease. *J. Rheumatol.* 1993;20:838–44.

[48] Maas D, Schramm A, Jackle B, RaifW, Schubothe H. Progressive systemic sclerosis — long-termtreatmentwith azathioprin (author's transl).*Immun. Infekt.* 1979;7:165–9.

[49] Nadashkevich O, Davis P, Fritzler M, Kovalenko W. A randomized unblinded trial of cyclophosphamide versus azathioprine in the treatment of systemic sclerosis. *Clin. Rheumatol.* 2006; 25(2):205–12. [PubMed: 16228107]

[50] Berezne A, Ranque B, Valeyre D, et al. Therapeutic strategy combining intravenous cyclophosphamide followed by oral azathioprine to treat worsening interstitial lung disease associated with systemic sclerosis: a retrospective multicenter open-label study. *J. Rheumatol.* 2008; 35(6):1064–72. [PubMed: 18464307]

[51] Stratton RJ, Wilson H, Black CM. Pilot study of anti-thymocyte globulin plus mycophenolate mofetil in recent-onset diffuse scleroderma. *Rheumatology* (Oxford). 2001; 40(1):84–8. [PubMed: 11157146]

[52] Swigris JJ, Olson AL, Fischer A, et al. Mycophenolate mofetil is safe, well tolerated, and preserves lung function in patients with connective tissue disease-related interstitial lung disease. *Chest.* 2006; 130(1):30–6. [PubMed: 16840379]

[53] Liossis SN, Bounas A, Andonopoulos AP. Mycophenolate mofetil as first-line treatment improves clinically evident early scleroderma lung disease. *Rheumatology* (Oxford). 2006; 45(8): 1005–8. [PubMed: 16490756]

[54] Zamora AC, Wolters PJ, Collard HR, et al. Use of mycophenolate mofetil to treat sclerodermaassociated interstitial lung disease. *Respir. Med.* 2008; 102(1):150–5. [PubMed: 17822892]

[55] Gerbino AJ, Goss CH, Molitor JA. Effect of mycophenolate mofetil on pulmonary function in scleroderma-associated interstitial lung disease. *Chest.* 2008; 133(2):455–60. [PubMed: 18071023]

[56] Nihtyanova SI, Brough GM, Black CM, Denton CP. Mycophenolate mofetil in diffuse cutaneous systemic sclerosis—a retrospective analysis. *Rheumatology* (Oxford) 2007;46:442–5.

[57] Pope JE, Bellamy N, Seibold JR, Baron M, Ellman M, Carette S, Smith CD, Chalmers IM, Hong P, O'Hanlon D, Kaminska E, Markland J, Sibley J, Catoggio L, Furst DE. A randomized, controlled trial of methotrexate versus placebo in early diffuse scleroderma. *Arthritis Rheum.* 2001 Jun;44(6):1351.

[58] Van den Hoogen FH, Boerbooms AM, Swaak AJ, Rasker JJ, van Lier HJ, van de Putte LB. Comparison of methotrexate with placebo in the treatment of systemic sclerosis: a 24 week randomized double-blind trial, followed by a 24 week observational trial. *Br. J. Rheumatol.* 1996 Apr;35(4):364-72.

[59] Seibold JR, Denton CP, Furst DE, Guillevin L, Rubin LJ, Wells A, Matucci Cerinic M, Riemekasten G, Emery P, Chadha-Boreham H, Charef P, Roux S, Black CM. Arthritis Rheum. 2010 Jul;62(7):2101-8. doi: 10.1002/art.27466. Erratum in: *Arthritis Rheum.* 2010 Oct;62(10):3005.

[60] Buch MH, Denton CP, Furst DE, Guillevin L, Rubin LJ, Wells AU, Matucci-Cerinic M, Riemekasten G, Emery P, Chadha-Boreham H, Charef P, Roux S, Black CM, Seibold JR.Ann Rheum Dis. Submaximal exercise testing in the assessment of interstitial lung disease secondary to

systemic sclerosis: reproducibility and correlations of the 6-min walk test. 2007 Feb;66(2):169-73. Epub 2006 Jul 25.

[61] BUILD-1: a randomized placebo-controlled trial of bosentan in idiopathic pulmonary fibrosis. King TE Jr, Behr J, Brown KK, du Bois RM, Lancaster L, de Andrade JA, Stähler G, Leconte I, Roux S, Raghu G. *Am. J. Respir. Crit. Care Med.* 2008 Jan 1;177(1):75-81. Epub 2007 Sep 27.

[62] King TE Jr, Brown KK, Raghu G, du Bois RM, Lynch DA, Martinez F, Valeyre D, Leconte I, Morganti A, Roux S, Behr J. *Am. J. Respir. Crit. Care Med.* BUILD-3: a randomized, controlled trial of bosentan in idiopathic pulmonary fibrosis. 2011 Jul 1;184(1):92-9. doi: 10.1164/rccm.201011-1874OC. Epub 2011 Apr 7.

[63] Akhmetshina A, Venalis P, Dees C, Busch N, Zwerina J, Schett G. Treatment with imatinib prevents fibrosis in different preclinical models of systemic sclerosis and induces regression of established fibrosis. *Arthritis and Rheumatism* 2009;60:219–24.

[64] Ghofrani HA, Seeger W, Grimminger F. Imatinib for the treatment of pulmonary arterial hypertension. *The New England Journal of Medicine* 2005;353:1412–3.

[65] Distler JH, Manger B, Spriewald BM, Schett G, Distler O. Treatment of pulmonary fibrosis for twenty weeks with imatinib mesylate in a patient with mixed connective tissue disease. *Arthritis and Rheumatism* 2008;58:2538–42.

[66] Sabnani I, Zucker MJ, Rosenstein ED, Baran DA, Arroyo LH, Tsang P, et al. A novel therapeutic approach to the treatment of scleroderma-associated pulmonary complications: safety and efficacy of combination therapy with imatinib and cyclophosphamide. *Rheumatology* (Oxford) 2009;48:49–52.

[67] Khanna D, Saggar R, Mayes MD, Abtin F, Clements PJ, Maranian P, Assassi S, Saggar R, Singh RR, Furst DE.Arthritis Rheum. A one-year, phase I/IIa, open-label pilot trial of imatinib mesylate in the treatment of systemic sclerosis-associated active interstitial lung disease. 2011 Nov;63(11):3540-6. doi: 10.1002/art.30548.

[68] Akhmetshina A, Dees C, Pileckyte M, Maurer B, Axmann R, Jüngel A, Zwerina J, Gay S, Schett G, Distler O, Distler JH. Dual inhibition of c-abl and PDGF receptor signaling by dasatinib and nilotinib for the treatment of dermal fibrosis. *FASEB J.* 2008 Jul;22(7):2214-22. doi: 10.1096/fj.07-105627. Epub 2008 Mar 7.

[69] Richter A, Puddicombe SM, Lordan JL, Bucchieri F, Wilson SJ, Djukanovic R, Dent G, Holgate ST, Davies DE. The contribution of interleukin (IL)-4 and IL-13 to the epithelial-mesenchymal trophic unit in asthma. *Am. J. Respir. Cell Mol. Biol.* 2001 Sep;25(3):385-91.

[70] Hasegawa M, Fujimoto M, Kikuchi K, Takehara K. J. Elevated serum levels of interleukin 4 (IL-4), IL-10, and IL-13 in patients with systemic sclerosis. *Rheumatol.* 1997 Feb;24(2):328-32.

[71] Riccieri V, Rinaldi T, Spadaro A, Scrivo R, Ceccarelli F, Franco MD, Taccari E, Valesini G. Interleukin-13 in systemic sclerosis: relationship to nailfold capillaroscopy abnormalities. *Clin. Rheumatol.* 2003 May;22(2):102-6.

[72] Zhu Z, Homer RJ, Wang Z, Chen Q, Geba GP, Wang J, Zhang Y, Elias JA. Pulmonary expression of interleukin-13 causes inflammation, mucus hypersecretion, subepithelial fibrosis, physiologic abnormalities, and eotaxin production. *J. Clin. Invest.* 1999 Mar;103(6):779-88.

[73] Liu T, Jin H, Ullenbruch M, Hu B, Hashimoto N, Moore B, McKenzie A, Lukacs NW, Phan SH. Regulation of found in inflammatory zone 1 expression in bleomycin-induced lung fibrosis: role of IL-4/IL-13 and mediation via STAT-6. *J. Immunol.* 2004 Sep 1;173(5):3425-31.

[74] Jakubzick C, Choi ES, Joshi BH, Keane MP, Kunkel SL, Puri RK, Hogaboam CM.J Immunol. 2003 Sep 1;171(5):2684-93.Therapeutic attenuation of pulmonary fibrosis via targeting of IL-4- and IL-13-responsive cells.

[75] Sato S, Hasegawa M, Takehara K. Serum levels of interleukin-6 and interleukin-10 correlate with total skin thickness score in patients with systemic sclerosis. *Journal of Dermatological Science* 2001;27:140–6.

[76] De Lauretis A, Sestini P, Pantelidis P, Hoyles R, Hansell DM, Goh NS, Zappala CJ, Visca D, Maher TM, Denton CP, Ong VH, Abraham DJ, Kelleher P, Hector L, Wells AU, Renzoni EA. Serum Interleukin 6 Is Predictive of Early Functional Decline and Mortality in Interstitial Lung Disease Associated with Systemic Sclerosis, *J. Rheumatol.* 2013 Feb 1. [Epub ahead of print]

[77] Saito F, Tasaka S, Inoue K, Miyamoto K, Nakano Y, Ogawa Y, et al. Role of interleukin-6 in bleomycin-induced lung inflammatory changes in mice. *American Journal of Respiratory Cell and Molecular Biology* 2008;38:566–71.

[78] Shima Y, Kuwahara Y, Murota H, Kitaba S, Kawai M, Hirano T, et al. The skin of patients with systemic sclerosis softened during the

treatment with anti-IL-6 receptor antibody tocilizumab. *Rheumatology* 2010;49:2408–12.

[79] Lafyatis R, O'Hara C, Feghali-Bostwick CA, Matteson E. B cell infiltration in systemic sclerosis-associated interstitial lung disease. *Arthritis Rheum.* 2007 Sep;56(9):3167-8. No abstract available.

[80] Hasegawa M, Hamaguchi Y, Yanaba K, Bouaziz JD, Uchida J, Fujimoto M, Matsushita T, Matsushita Y, Horikawa M, Komura K, Takehara K, Sato S, Tedder TF. B-lymphocyte depletion reduces skin fibrosis and autoimmunity in the tight-skin mouse model for systemic sclerosis. *Am. J. Pathol.* 2006 Sep;169(3):954-66.

[81] McGonagle D, Tan AL, Madden J, Rawstron AC, Rehman A, Emery P, et al. Successful treatment of resistant scleroderma-associated interstitial lung disease with rituximab. *Rheumatology* (Oxford) 2008;47:552–3.

[82] Daoussis D, Liossis SN, Tsamandas AC, Kalogeropoulou C, Kazantzi A, Korfiatis P, et al. Is there a role for b-cell depletion as therapy for scleroderma? A case report and review of the literature. *Semin Arthritis Rheum.* 2009 Dec 9.

[83] Daoussis D, Liossis SN, Tsamandas AC, Kalogeropoulou C, Kazantzi A, Sirinian C, et al. Experience with rituximab in scleroderma: results from a 1-year, proof-of principle study. *Rheumatology* (Oxford) 2010;49:271–80.

[84] Demedts M, Behr J, Buhl R, Costabel U, Dekhuijzen R, Jansen HM, et al. High-dose acetylcysteine in idiopathic pulmonary fibrosis. *N. Engl. J. Med.* 2005;353:2229–42.

[85] Rosato E, Rossi C, Molinaro I, Giovannetti A, Pisarri S, Salsano F. Long-term N-acetylcysteine therapy in systemic sclerosis interstitial lung disease: a retrospective study. *Int. J. Immunopathol. Pharmacol.* 2011 Jul-Sep;24(3):727-33.

[86] Cipriani P, Carubbi F, Liakouli V, Marrelli A, Perricone C, Perricone R, Alesse E, Giacomelli R. Stem cells in autoimmune diseases: Implications for pathogenesis and future trends in therapy. *Autoimmun. Rev.* 2012 Nov 24. doi:pii: S1568-9972(12)00262-5. 10.1016/j.autrev. 2012.10.004. [Epub ahead of print]

[87] Burt RK, Shah SJ, Dill K, Grant T, Gheorghiade M, Schroeder J, Craig R, Hirano I, Marshall K, Ruderman E, Jovanovic B, Milanetti F, Jain S, Boyce K, Morgan A, Carr J, Barr W. Autologous non-myeloablative haemopoietic stem-cell transplantation compared with pulse cyclophosphamide once per month for systemic sclerosis (ASSIST): an

open-label, randomised phase 2 trial. *Lancet.* 2011 Aug 6;378 (9790): 498-506. doi: 10.1016/S0140-6736(11)60982-3. Epub 2011 Jul 21.

[88]   Rojas M, Xu J, Woods CR, Mora AL, Spears W, Roman J, Brigham KL. Bone marrow-derived mesenchymal stem cells in repair of the injured lung. *Am. J. Respir. Cell Mol. Biol.* 2005 Aug;33(2):145-52. Epub 2005 May 12.

[89]   Zhao F, Zhang YF, Liu YG, Zhou JJ, Li ZK, Wu CG, Qi HW. Therapeutic effects of bone marrow-derived mesenchymal stem cells engraftment on bleomycin-induced lung injury in rats. *Transplant Proc.* 2008 Jun;40(5):1700-5. doi: 10.1016/j.transproceed.2008.01.080.

[90]   Serrano-Mollar A, Nacher M, Gay-Jordi G, Closa D, Xaubet A, Bulbena O.Am J Respir Crit Care Med. Intratracheal transplantation of alveolar type II cells reverses bleomycin-induced lung fibrosis. 2007 Dec 15;176(12):1261-8. Epub 2007 Jul 19.

[91]   Schachna L, Medsger TA Jr, Dauber JH, Wigley FM, Braunstein NA, White B, et al. Lung transplantation in scleroderma compared with idiopathic pulmonary fibrosis and idiopathic pulmonary arterial hypertension. *Arthritis Rheum.* 2006; 54:3954–61.

[92]   Saggar R, Khanna D, Furst DE, Belperio JA, Park GS, Weigt SS, et al. Systemic sclerosis and bilateral lung transplantation: a single center experience. *Eur. Respir. J.* 2010; 36:893–900.

[93]   Shitrit D, Amital A, Peled N, et al. Lung transplantation in patients with scleroderma: case series, review of the literature, and criteria for transplantation. *Clin. Transplant.* 2009; 23(2):178–83.

In: Scleroderma
Editor: Romain De Winter

ISBN: 978-1-62618-802-0
© 2013 Nova Science Publishers, Inc.

Chapter III

Nailfold Capillaroscopy and Early Diagnosis of Systemic Sclerosis

Slavica Pavlov-Dolijanovic[1]
and Nada Vujasinovic Stupar[2]
[1]Institute of Rheumatology Belgrade, Serbia
[2]Faculty of Medicine University of Belgrade,
Institute of Rheumatology, Serbia

Abstract

Nailfold capillaroscopy is an essential imaging technique and the best method to analyse microvascular abnormalities in autoimmune rheumatic diseases. Capillary microscopy seems to be a useful tool for early selection of those patients who are potentially candidates for developing scleroderma spectrum disorders, especially systemic sclerosis (SSc). Architectural disorganization, giant capillaries, haemorrhages, loss of capillaries, angiogenesis and avascular areas characterize >90% of patients with overt SSc. The term "SSc pattern" includes, all together, these sequential capillaroscopic changes typical to the microvascular involvement in SSc. Three different patterns identified within the "SSc pattern"-early, active and late. Several different laboratory variables (serum E-selectin, serum tissue kallikrein, plasma endothelin 1, homocystein, urinary metabolites of F2-isoprostanes, serum anti-endothelial cell antibodies, antitopoisomerase I antibodies, anticentromere antibodies, anti-CENP-B, anti Th/To antibodies and anti-RNAP III) and clinical manifestations in SSc (peripheral vascular, skin, and lung involvement) have been shown to be associated with different pattern of capillary abnormality, providing further insights into disease pathogenesis.

Keywords: Nailfold capillaroscopy, systemic sclerosis, early diagnosis

Nailfold capillaroscopy (NFC) is an essential imaging technique for the in vivo assessment of microcirculation [1-4] and one of the best diagnostic tools for the early detection of systemic sclerosis (SSc) [5]. Generally, NFC is performed by means of a series of instruments, including the ophthalmoscope, the stereomicroscope [6], handheld dermatoscope [7], and more recently, video capillaroscopic system [8] (Figure 1). The last one in comparison with the older wide field technique has a high magnification (200-600x compared with 12-14x).

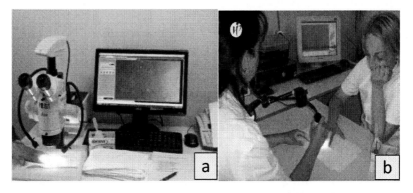

Figure 1. The present nailfold copillaroscope in author's hospital: a) Leica stereo microscope with a halogen light source (Leica MZ 95, KL 1500LCD, Germany) and b) nailfold videocapillaroscope analysis (Videocap, DS MediGroup, Italy).

Standard Technique
for Capillaroscopic Examination

The study of NFC in patients with rheumatic disorders analyzes the nailfold skin of hands (Figure 2). This area is easily accessible for examination, and here the major axis of the capillaries is parallel to the skin surface, whereas in other skin areas, the capillaries run perpendicular to the skin surface.

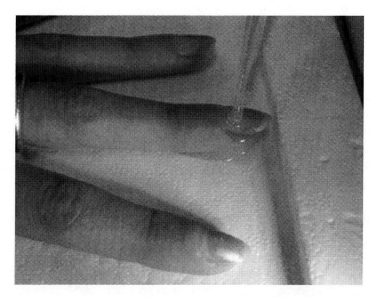

Figure 2. A drop of immersion oil is placed on the nailfold bed to improve resolution.

Ideally, patients should be seated indoors for a minimum of 15 minutes before the nailfold analysis can be performed, to acclimatize to the room temperature of 20-24^{0}C. The nailfolds in each finger should be examined. Fingers affected by recent trauma are not analyzed. To improve the image resolution, a drop of immersion oil is placed on the nailfold bed. Cedar or paraffin oil is the preferable as immersion oil due to its higher viscosity.

Clinical Implications from Capillaroscopy

According to the the literature data, capillaroscopy should be carried out on all patients affected by Raunaud's phenomenon (RP). RP is seen in 5-10% of the population and generally follows an indolent course. It can be classified as a primary RP of unknown cause, or as a secondary one related to a number of different diseases, including connective tissue diseases (CTDs) [9, 10]. Very recently, in follow-up study of 3035 patients with initially rigorously defined as primary RP, who sought for consultation with rheumatologist in tertiary care hospital, noticed the development of associated CTDs in 37.2% of suffers, during the mean follow-up of 4.3 years. The mean time interval between beginning of RP and the development of CTDs was 6.2 years. A spectrum of 12 different underlying diseases was recorded. The most frequently were recorded undifferentiated CTD (~12%) and SSc (~9%). The followed: systemic lupus erythematosus (SLE) (4.7%), rheumatoid arthritis (3.5%), scleroderma overlap syndrome (3.4%), Sjögren's syndrome (2%) and less than 1% of patients developed systemic vasculitis, polymyositis /dermatomyositis, mixed connective tissue disease, primary antiphospholipid syndrome, psoriatic arthritis or ankylosing spondylitis [11].

For the reason of prognosis, early diagnosis, and better treatment results, it is important to know which patients with RP will develop or are already evolving into a CTD, especially SSc. The European League Against Rheumatism (EULAR) Scleroderma Trial and Research Group proposed another set of criteria for very early diagnosis of SSc [12].

According to this recommendations either all 3 major criteria (RP, the presence of antibodies [antinuclear, anticentromere, antitopoisomerase I], and abnormal results of diagnostic NFC), or 2 major and 1 additional criteria (calcinosis, puffy fingers, digital ulcers, dysfunction of the oesophageal sphincter, telangiectasia and ground-glass on the chest high-resolution computed tomography) must be met.

Although these criteria require one other abnormal clinical or laboratory feature in addition to abnormal results of NFC for a diagnosis of SSc in RP patients, nonetheless they support a central role of NFC in the identification of early SSc. Moreover, capillaroscopy examination should be performed in patients with morphea [7] and suspected eosinophilic fasciitis [13], characterized by a normal capillaroscopic picture. Therefore, the presence of morphologic abnormalities ranging in the scleroderma pattern should exclude the diagnosis of a localized form of CTD.

Capillaroscopic Microvascular Morphology

During capillaroscopic examination, the following microvascular morphology should be observed: capillary morphology, loop size, density, capillary loss, angiogenesis, microhemorrhage, and subpapillary venous plexus.

Capillary Morphology

In healthy subjects, capillary morphology is "reverse U-shaped" or "hairpin-like" in appearance (Figure 3). Tortuosity is usually a physiological variation that refers to an irregular or undulating appearance with single/multiple crossover (Figure 4). Tortuosity has limited diagnostic value but more frequently it could be registered in SLE patients [14], and may indicate angiogenesis in some diseases [15].

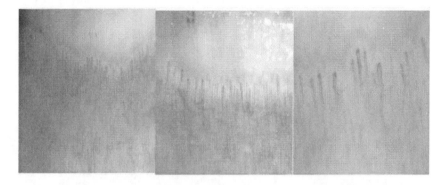

Figure 3. The normal nailfold capillaroscope pattern, showing the regular disposition of the capillary loops along with the nail bed without dilatation and capillary loss in a healthy subjects (sequential magnifications x50, x100, x200).

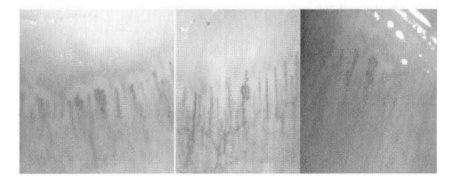

Figure 4. Tortuous (irregular or undulating appearance with single/multiple crossover) and bushy (several buds are observed sprouting out) capillary loops.

Loop Size

The average length of capillary loop is 475 μm, and a length exceeding 700 μm is defined as loop elongation. The capillary length of the fourth and fifth fingers is always longer than that of the other fingers [16]. The diameter of the afferent (arterial) limb capillary can vary from 6 to19 μm (mean value: 11 ± 3 μm) and the diameter of the efferent (venous) limb is 8-20 μm (mean value: 12 ± 3 μm) [17]. The efferent limb is usually of greater diameter than the afferent limb, but the venous: arterial limb diameter ratio does not exceed 2:1 [16] (Figure 5).

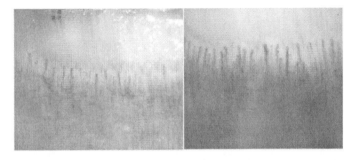

Figure 5. Capillary morphological anomalies with homogeneously dilated efferent limb in sequentian magnifications (x50, x100). Normal (typical) capillary loop looks hairpin.

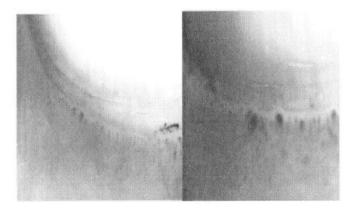

Figure 6. Presence of microhemorrhage, enlarged and giant (megacapillaries) capillary loops.

Enlarged capillaries are characterized by a 4-fold increase in the size or capillary diameter exceeding 20 μm. Additionally, capillaries with a 10-fold larger diameter than the normal range or more than 50 μm are referred to a giant capillaries or megacapillaries (Figure 6) [5, 16-19]. Even the detection of a single loop with a circumscribed or homogeneous diameter >50 should be considered as a potential marker of microangiopathy related to an early scleroderma-spectrum disorder [18].

Density

At the nailfold, each dermal papilla has 1 to 3 capillaries (Figure 7). Six to 14 capillaries per millimeter or 10 to 30 capillaries per square millimeter are visible. It is called normal density [19].

Figure 7. Miscoscopic image of nailfold with normal capillary density: each dermapapilla has 1 to 3 capillaries.

Loss of Capillaries (Avascular Areas)

A decrease number of loops (<30 over 5mm length in the distal row of the nailfold) or loss of capillaries in a field of at least 500 μm should be considered an avascular area (Figure 8). This pattern is highly persistent characteristic of SSc and has been associated with more extensive skin involvement and a poor prognosis [20]. Loss of capillaries and enlarged or giant capillaries may be represents a local autoregulatory response to tissue hypoxia.

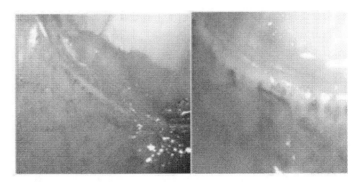

Figure 8. Presence of avascular areas.

Angiogenesis

Capillary neoformation (angiogenesis) may be also related to tissue hypoxia (Figure 9). The features of capillary neoformation may be very heterogeneous: (1) extremely tortuous, branching, "bushy" (ramified) and "coiled" capillaries; (2) more than 4 capillaries with dermal papilla; (3) extremely elongated loops; and (4) thin, branching, and interconnected capillaries [21].

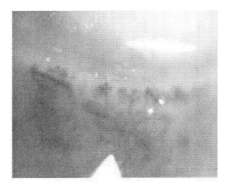

Figure 9. Presence of angiogenesis. An artificial light reflex is noted near the nailfold.

Microhaemorrhage

Local microhaemorrhages (microbleeding) are also associated with early vascular damage and it appears as an easily detectable dark spot (Figure 10).

These were classified according to their distribution pattern as focal or diffuse, when grouped within limited areas or distributed throughout the periungal region respectively. Capillary thrombosis may be misinterpreted as microhaemorrhage. A prominent feature of thrombosis is the shape of the dark area, which mirrors that of the capillary loop [19].

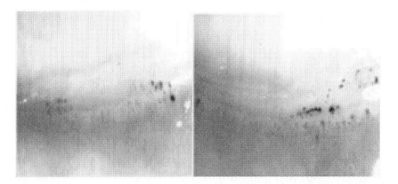

Figure 10. Microhaermorrhages are almost always observed in the typical patterns of the connective tissue diseases.

Subpapillary Venous Plexus

The deep arterial plexus connects with superficial vessels and finally with terminal arterioles, which begin the afferent limb of the capillary loops. The efferent limb merges with the superficial subpapillary venous plexus and intercommunicates with deep venous plexuses (Figure 11). The subpapillary venous plexus is visible in approximately one-third of healthy humans [16].

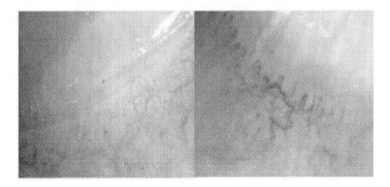

Figure 11. Presence of subpapilary venous plexus.

Normal versus Abnormal Finding in Nailfold Capillaroscopy

A theoretically the normal capillary pattern of the distal capillaries row of the nailfold included an open hairpin shape, homogenous size, regularly arranged in a parallel fashion, with mean number of 9 per mm (ranged from 6 to 14). This reference, however, cannot be considered as representative because of findings of wide variations in the ranges of the normal morphology across the population. Andrade et al. [22] reported capillaroscopic findings on the largest (N= 800) described healthy persons study population. Morphological anomalies were seen in 34% of healthy persons, but few in each individual. Unusual distinctive capillary alterations were: meandering loops (limbs crossed upon themselves or with another several times) in 25%, ectatic loops (afferent, transition and efferent limbs are moderately enlarged) in 12%, bushy loops (the limbs originate small and result in multiple buds) in 7% and bizarre loops (striking atypical morphology, but not classifiable in the previous categories) in 2%. Giant capillaries or extensive avascularity have not been detected in a normal population and should be considered as pathological.

Age Related Findings of Nailfold Capillaroscopy

The normal nailfold capillary network in children resembles that observed in adults with some differences, such as a lower number of loops per millimeter (five to nine), a higher plexus visualization score, and a higher frequency of atypical loops (meandering, enlarged, bushy, and bizarre capillaries). This is important information because devascularization is one of the major objective signs of scleroderma microangiopathy. Bizarre capillaries (open-ended spanner loop) represent a distinct feature of children's capillary network, because they are not usually observed in normal adults. Only in children older 10 years of age, capillary morphology was similar to that in adults [23]. These differences should ideally be age adjusted, and loop size should not be categorized as normal or abnormal without taking the child's age into account [24].

In subjects over the age of 70 enlargement of nailfold capillaries and a prominent subpapillary venous plexus are observed. Enlargement and congestion of venules and capillaries seem to be related to the permanent opening of arteriovenous anastomoses, and belong to "senile microangiopathy" [25].

Today, there is a general consensus between experts in defining the normal range as decisively vast and varied enough to be able to be paradoxically considered characterized by the absence of expressions of a clearly evident pathology [26].

Scleroderma Pattern of Nailfold Capillaroscopy

The majority of patients with clinically recognizable SSc show a very characteristic combination of capillary abnormalities (architectural disorganization, enlarged loops, loss of capillaries, hemorrhages, angiogenesis and avascular areas), the "scleroderma-type" changes, which can easily be assessed through pattern recognition [1, 21]. Since the morphological markers of the microvasculature damage in SSc are dynamic and progressive, these have been recently reclassified by Cutolo et al. [8] into 3 defined and different NFC patterns that include an early, active or late pattern. An "early" pattern (few enlarged/giant capillaries, few capillary hemorrhages, relatively well-preserved capillary distribution and no evident loss of capillaries), an "active" pattern (frequent giant capillaries, frequent capillary hemorrhages, moderate loss of capillaries, mild disorganization of the capillary architecture and absent or mild ramified capillaries), and a "late" pattern (almost absent giant capillaries and microhemorrhages, severe loss of capillaries with extensive avascular areas, ramified/bushy capillaries, and intense disorganization of the normal capillary array) (Figure 12).

In particular, the detection of enlarged and giant capillaries, together with microextravasation of the red blood cells (hemorrhage) in the nailfold, most likely represents the first, initial morphologic sign of the altered micro-circulation in SSc. The early stage is also characterized by microvessels with a normal diameter coexisting with a few enlarged capillaries [27]. We have to carefully investigate all fingers by considering the limited number of these nailfold changes during early phases of the disease. Conversely, these changes are strongly increased in SSc patients with an "active" pattern. As the pathophysiologic process of SSc progress into fibrotic phase of the disease, the capillaroscopy analysis most likely reflects the effects of tissue hypoxia: massive capillary destruction, loss of capillaries, together with vascular architectural disorganisation and ramified capillaries indicating neoangiogenesis. This advanced stage of SSc is characterized by the late capillaroscopic pattern [8]. These capillaroscopic patterns are descriptive and there is inevitable overlap between them.

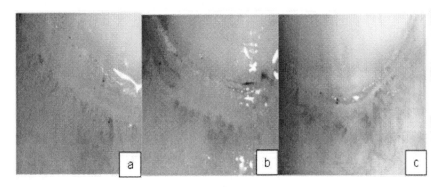

Figure 12. The three different scleroderma patterns can be seen here: early (a), active (b), and late (c).

Sulli et al. [28] indicated to examine changes in patterns over time. Also, in patients with RP associated with SSc-spectrum disorders morphological features of the nailfold microvascular bed may show a higher degree of morphological variability, even after few days. On the contrary, in healthy control subjects as well as in patients with primary RP the capillaroscopic pattern may remain unchanged for a long time.

Nailfold Capillaroscopy and Early Diagnosis of SSc

Capillaroscopic observation, even in childhood rheumatic diseases and healthy controls, have confirmed their usefulness in early recognition and monitoring scleroderma spectrum disorders [29].

Children and adolescent with RP who developed scleroderma spectrum disorders showed a sclerodermatous type of capillary changes 6 months before the expression of the disease, indicating that this type of capillary changes in children and adolescents with RP highly correlated with future development of scleroderma spectrum disorders [30]. In addition, in childhood RP, nailfold capillaroscopy is a non-invasive examination enabling early diagnosis of "systemic scleroderma sine scleroderma" [31].

Preliminary data from the EULAR Scleroderma Trial and Research group (EUSTAR) database [32] indicate the mean time between the onset of RP and the first non-RP symptoms or signs in SSc is 4.8 years in limited cutaneous SSc in contrast to 1.9 years in diffuse cutaneous SSc. Matucci-Cerinic et al. [12] considered that this time gap between symptoms and diagnosis, mainly based on dermal or internal organ fibrosis, could be regarded as a *"window of opportunity"* for SSc, and therefore should be future target for all investigators. These authors proposed that RP, disease-specific autoantibodies (antinuclear, anticentromere, antitopoisomerase I), and pathognomotic microvascular alteration detected by capillaroscopy may represent the three corners of "triangle", defining true "prescleroderma" phase before skin becomes really involved. These parameters composite pyramid whose key to very early SSc still needs to be identified. Puffy fingers are presented in the centre of this pyramid as a sign presented in mixed CTD, undifferentiated CTD and prescleroderma (*"presclerodermatous"* disease).

More recently, after 3 Delphi rounds seeking expert opinion criteria for very early SSc and categorizing of their 23 items, it was suggested that abnormal capillaroscopy with scleroderma pattern ranked highest in the final list together with RP, SSc-specific autoantibodies, and the presence of skin thickening [33].

Johnson et al. [34] evaluated face validity of potential classification criteria for SSc using the frequency of items in patients with SSc (N= 783) and those with diseases similar to SSc (mimickers, N= 1071): systemic lupus erythematosus (N= 499), myositis (N= 171), Sjogren's syndrome (N= 95), RP (N= 228), mixed CTD (N= 29), and idiopathic pulmonary arterial hypertension (N= 49). Discriminated validity was evaluated using odds ratios (ORs). Compared to mimickers, patients with SSc among other items were more likely to have puffy fingers (OR 35), anti-topoisomerase I antibody (OR 25), RP (OR 24), anticentromere antibody (OR 14), abnormal nailfold capillaries (OR 10), and antinuclear antibody (OR 6).

Also, very recently, in a prospective outcome study with mean follow-up of 4,8 years (range 1-10 years), nailfold scleroderma pattern abnormalities were confirmed to have a prognostic valuae in RP patients. The nailfold capillaroscopic morphological aspect was analyzed in 3029 patients initially referred as affected by primary RP. SSc pattern was significantly associated with the development of SSc (sensitivity 94%, specificity 92%, positive predictive valuae 52%, negative predictive valuae 99% and OR 163), as well as dermatomyositis (OR 13.67), overlap syndrome with signs of SSc (OR 4.83) and mixed CTD (OR 3.3) [35[. Clearly, all these investigations over the last decade have increased the interest and need for capillaroscopy, at least in the early diagnosis of SSc [36].

Capillaroscopic Analysis, Serological Abnormalities and Laboratory Markers in SSc

SSc is characterized by serum autoantibodies, including anticentromere (ACA), anti-Th/To, anti-topoisomerase I (anti-Scl70), and anti/RNA polymerase I/III (anti RNAP III). Together, these markers account for almost 85% of autoantibodies specific for SSc and show a predictive value for clinical evaluation and prognosis [37, 38]. Many studies indicate that these autoantibodies may be important factors associated with qualitative and quantitative capillaroscopic changes, whereas there is no clear explanation of this association.

Some authors have linked the presence of ACA to a capillaroscopic pattern with a predominance of capillary enlargement [4, 20, 21], whilst the presence of anti-Scl70 antibodies was significantly associated with the avascular areas [39]. Cutolo et al. [40] showed that anti-Scl70 antibodies seems be related to earlier expression of the "active" and "late" NFC patterns of SSc microvascular damage, while the presence of ACA seems to be related to delayed expression of the "late" NFC pattern.

Koenig et al. [41] reported that enlarged/giant capillaries, capillary loss, and SSc-specific autoantibodies independently predicted definite SSc. Interestingly, ACA and anti-Th/To antibodies predicted for the development of enlarged capillaries; these autoantibodies and anti-RNAP III predicted for capillary loss. Each autoantibody was associated with a distinct time course of microvascular damage as caused by capillary enlargement or capillary loss. At follow-up, 79.5% of patients with one of these autoantibodies and abnormal NFC findings at baseline had developed definite SSc. Patients with both baseline predictors, namely abnormal capillaroscopy and an SSc-specific autoantibody were 60 times more likely to develop definite SSc. These data validated the proposed criteria for early SSc. In conclusion, in the presence of a secondary RP evolving to definite SSc, microvascular damage (as assessed by NFC) is dynamic and progressive, and SSc-specific autoantibodies are associated with the course and type of capillary abnormalities. It was confirmed that the microvascular damage in secondary RP evolving to definitive SSc is characteristically sequential, starting with enlarged capillaries /giant capillaries ("early" SSc pattern), followed by capillary loss ("active" SSc pattern), and then by capillary telangiectasias (neoangiogenesis "late" SSc pattern) [42].

The several studies have investigated possible links between microvascular abnormalities and specific laboratory markers of SSc. One of the first one [43] showed a correlation between soluble serum E-selectin levels and alterations in capillaroscopy (capillary loss), especially in patients with early disease (within 48 months of diagnosis), suggesting that serum E-selectin levels might be a useful biochemical marker of disease activity in SSc. E-selectin is particularly interesting because it is found only on the activated endothelium in contrast to other adhesion molecules which have a wide tissue distribution.

Circulating levels of tissue kallikrein, acting on the microcirculation as a potent angiogenic agent, were higher in SSc patients with early and active capillaroscopic pattern than in those with late pattern [44]. Patients with giant capillaries and capillary microhaemorrhages had higher tissue kallikrein concentrations than those with architectural derangement suggesting that tissue kallikrein may play a part in SSc microvascular changes.

Endothelin 1 plays an important role in SSc by causing vascular endothelial cell proliferation, vasoconstriction, smooth muscle hypertrophy, irreversible vascular remodeling in the lungs, and by promoting fibroblast synthesis of type I and type III collagen and fibronectin by a receptor-dependent mechanism. Interestingly, detection the highest endothelin 1 plasma levels in the more advanced stage of the SSc microangiopathy, namely the "late" NFC pattern, characterized by capillary loss and increased tissue fibrosis seems to support the involvement of endothelin 1 in the progression from microvascular to fibrotic SSc damage [45].

Homocystein is a nonessential amino acid that interferes with normal properties of vascular tree. As know, hyperhomocysteinemia may cause vascular damage by several mechanisms: it is directly toxic to endothelium and may impair its physiological thromboresistance by interfering with the action of natural anticoagulant like protein C, thrombomodulin, and annexin II. Moreover, homocystein may favor an oxidant status by generating superoxide radicals, by inhibiting antioxidant enzymes, and supporting oxidation of low density lipoprotein by arterial smooth muscle cells. Finally, in vitro was demonstrated that homocystein alters nitric oxide release by cultured endothelial cells, and increases collagen production by cultured rabbit smooth muscle cells. Caramaschi et al. [46] showed that homocysteine plasma level is related to microvascular involvement in SSc patients. Homocystein concentration increases with the progression of the NFC pattern from "early" to "active", and above all to "late" pattern. In conclusion, hyperhomocysteinemia may represent an aggravating factor among the complex mechanisms involved in scleroderma damage contributing to the injury of endothelium.

Anti-endothelial cell antibodies (AECAs) are a heterogeneous class of antibodies whose role in the pathogenesis of autoimmune diseases with vascular involvement has been extensively studied and are present in the serum samples of many patients with SSc (22-86%) but are not SSc specific [47]. AECAs were also more frequently found in SSc patients with the "late" capillaroscopic pattern [48]. This data suggest that AECAs may have a role in the progression of the endothelial damage in SSc, and their presence, especially in high titers, should be considered as adjunctive risk factor for a more severe disease with higher skin scores and cardiovascular involvement. Another study evaluating urinary concentration of 8-isoprostaglandin-F2 alpha as a marker of oxidative stress in SSc patients, showed a strong correlation between a marker of free radical damage with both the severity of lung involvement and the "active" and "late" capillaroscopic patterns [49]. In summary, several different laboratory variables have been shown to be associated with different patterns of capillary abnormality, providing further insights into disease pathogenesis.

Capillaroscopy and Clinical Manifestations in SSc

In the last few years, many investigators have evaluated in SSc patients the association of NFC patterns with both demographic and clinical features. The correlation between capillaroscopic findings and duration of the SSc is controversial. According to Cutolo et al. [8], the progression of capillary loss is correlated with the duration of the SSc, RP and the patient's age. This correlation, even if documented by various authors, is not always evident. Caramaschi et al. [50] showed that patients with "late" NFC pattern were older, and had longer disease duration in comparison with those with "early" and "active" pattern, but the difference did not reach statistical significance. Grassi et al. [26] believed that enlarged capillary loops and architectural disorders without manifest avascular areas may be dominant in patients with disease duration of >30 years. On the contrary, avascular areas can constitute the first dramatic capillaroscopic findings in SSc, especially in male subjects with a very aggressive "early" onset. There is evidence that progression of skin, lung, heart and peripheral vascular involvement were all related to the worsening of microangiopathy as directly assessed by NFC [50]. As expected, a very strong correlation was found between "late" pattern, which is characterized by avascular areas, and digital ulcers, a severe manifestation of peripheral vascular involvement that heavily affects the quality of life. An association with trophic lesion and loss of capillaries, as assessed by semiquantitative scoring, has also been reported [51]. Recently, it was found that the diffuse cutaneous form of SSc with avascular areas on capillaroscopy represented, among other factors (e.g., increased interleukin-6) the major risk factor for digital ulcers development [52]. In patients with SSc skin ulcers present for both patients and physician a major management problem. An early detection of SSc patients who are at high risk of developing digital ulcers (Figure 13) might allow preventive treatment with reduction of morbidity and social costs. A quantitative capillaroscopic score was suggested as highly predictive of the development of new skin digital ulcers within the first 3 months from NFC evaluation [53].

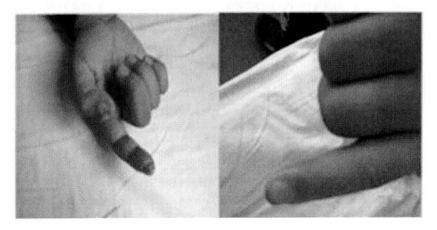

Figure 13. Classical skin digital ulcer in a patient affected by systemic sclerosis before and after treatment.

Alivernini et al. [52] reported that skin ulcers were present simultaneously with other vascular comorbidities, such as the reduction of TLCO, the presence of pulmonary arterial hypertension (PAH), a higher interstitial lung score, a history of arrhythmias, and the presence of heart block signs, which suggests that these lesion could be part of systemic process mainly characterized by endothelial damage.

They also showed that the occurrence of skin ulcers are more frequent in patients with diffuse skin involvement who have a higher Rodnan skin score, a higher positivity of anti Scl-70 autoantibody, antiphospholipid antibody, higher plasma level of IL-6, and the presence of NFC avascular areas. These results could be useful for the physician in daily practice to identify SSc patients with a higher risk of developing skin ulcers during the course of the disease.

Regarding the predictive value of capillaroscopy in visceral involvement, a study from 2004 showed that the association between ground-glass lung opacities and higher capillaroscopic avascular scores was particularly strong in SSc patients with disease duration of ≤ 5years [54]. In particular, ground-glass opacities were predominantly present in patients with advanced capillaroscopic alterations, but were absent in all patients with mild or without capillaroscopic alterations.

Therefore, NFC abnormalities might also reflect what is going on the pulmonary circulation. This may not be true for all capillary abnormalities, because most SSc patients demonstrate nailfold capillary abnormalities whereas only a minority develops PAH [42]. Recent study suggests that only capillary density reduction is a marker of the presence and severity of PAH. Capillary density was lower in SSc- PAH patients compared with SSc-nonPAH [55, 56], but loop dimensions were equal [55]. In comparison with idiopathic PAH, SSc-PAH patients had also reduced capillary density and larger loop dimensions. Capillary density in healthy subjects was significantly higher than in SSc patients with or without PAH, and patients with idiopathic PAH. Interestingly, capillary density negatively correlated with mean pulmonary arterial pressure at rest in SSc-PAH patients as well as in those with idiopathic PAH [55].

In contrast, Greidinger et al. [57] using capillary density and qualitative scoring of nailfold patterns, found no differences in capillary patterns between 8 patients with SSc-non-PAH and 7 with SSc-PAH, but capillary density in these groups was not reported. In conclusion, most of investigators [20, 58, 59] agree that the reduction in the number of capillaries with the appearance of avascular areas has a strongly indicative value with regards to the clinical variations of the illness characterized by an imprint denoting aggressiveness and rapid evolution.

Conclusion

Nailfold capillaroscopy is a best, simple, easy, safe, noninvasive, inexpensive, repeatable and highly sensitive method for the early diagnosis of systemic sclerosis through the detection of specific microvascular alterations that allows distinguishing the primary from secondary Raynaud's phenomenon, as well as, later, the progression of the disease.

References

[1]   Maricq HR. Wide-field capillary microscopy. *Arthritis Rheum.* 1981; 24:1159-65.

[2]   Houtman PM, Kallenberg CG, Fidler V, Wouda AA. Diagnostic significance of nailfold capillary patterns in patients with Raynaud's phenomenon. An analysis of patterns discriminating patients with and without connective tissue disease. *J. Rheumatol.* 1986; 13:556-63.

[3]   Statham BN, Rowell NR. Quantification of the nail fold capillary abnormalities in systemic sclerosis and Raynaud's syndrome. *Acta Derm. Venereol.* 1986;66:139-43.

[4]   Carpentier PH, Maricq HR. Microvasculature in systemic sclerosis. *Rheum. Dis. Clin. North Am.* 1990;16:75-91.

[5]   Cutolo M, Pizzorni C, Sulli A. Capillaroscopy. *Best Pract. Res. Clin. Rheumatol.*2005; 19:437-52.

[6]   Anders HJ, Sigl T, Schattenkirchner M. Differentiation between primary and secondary Raynaud's phenomenon: a prospective study comparing nailfold capillaroscopy using an ophthalmoscope or stereomicroscope. *Ann. Rheum. Dis.* 2001;60:407-9.

[7]   Bergman R, Sharony L, Schapira D, Nahir MA, Balbir-Gurman A. The handheld dermatoscope as a nail-fold capillaroscopic instrument. *Arch. Dermatol.* 2003;139:1027-30.

[8]   Cutolo M, Sulli A, Pizzorni C, Accardo S. Nailfold videocapillaroscopy assessment of microvascular damage in systemic sclerosis. *J. Rheumatol.* 2000;27: 155-60.

[9]   Maricq HR, Weinrich MC, Keil JE, LeRoy EC. Prevalence of Raynaud phenomenon in the general population. A preliminary study by questionnaire. *J. Chronic Dis.* 1986;39:423-7.

[10] Kallenberg CG. Connective tissue disease in patients presenting with Raynaud's phenomenon alone. *Ann. Rheum. Dis.* 1991;50:666-7.

[11] Pavlov-Dolijanovic S, Damjanov NS, Vujasinovic Stupar NZ, Radunovic GL, Stojanovic RM, Babic D. Late appearance and exacerbation of primary Raynaud's phenomenon attacks can predict future development of connective tissue disease: a retrospective chart review of 3,035 patients. *Rheumatol. Int.* 2012 Jul 22. [Epub ahead of print].

[12] Matucci-Cerinic M, Allanore Y, Czirják L, Tyndall A, Müller-Ladner U, Denton C, et al. The challenge of early systemic sclerosis for the EULAR Scleroderma Trial and Research group (EUSTAR) community. It is time to cut the Gordian knot and develop a prevention or rescue strategy. *Ann. Rheum. Dis.* 2009;68:1377-80.

[13] Rozboril MB, Maricq HR, Rodnan GP, Jablonska S, Bole GG. Capillary microscopy in eosinophilic fasciitis. A comparison with systemic sclerosis. *Arthritis Rheum.* 1983;26:617-22.

[14] Pavlov-Dolijanovic S, Damjanov NS, Vujasinovic Stupar NZ, Marcetic DR, Sefik-Bukilica MN, Petrovic RR. Is there a difference in systemic lupus erythematosus with and without Raynaud's phenomenon? *Rheumatol. Int.* 2012 May 22. [Epub ahead of print].

[15] Hern S, Mortimer PS. In vivo quantification of microvessels in clinically uninvolved psoriatic skin and in normal skin. *Br. J. Dermatol.* 2007;156:1224-9.

[16] Grassi W. Basic findings in capillaroscopy. Grassi W, Del Medico P. Atlas of capillaroscopy. 1 st Ed, Italy, EDRA, 2004;10-25.

[17] Anderson ME, Allen PD, Moore T, Hillier V, Taylor CJ, Herrick AL. Computerized nailfold video capillaroscopy-a new tool for assessment of Raynaud's phenomenon. *J. Rheumatol.* 2005;32:841-8.

[18] Cutolo M, Sulli A, Secchi ME, Olivieri M, Pizzorni C. The contribution of capillaroscopy to the differential diagnosis of connective autoimmune diseases. *Best Pract. Res. Clin. Rheumatol.* 2007;21:1093-108.

[19] Lin KM, Cheng TT, Chen CJ. Clinical applications of nailfold capillaroscopy in different rheumatic diseases. *J. Intern. Med. Taiwan* 2009;20:238-47.

[20] Chen ZY, Silver RM, Ainsworth SK, Dobson RL, Rust P, Maricq HR. Association between fluorescent antinuclear antibodies, capillary

patterns, and clinical features in scleroderma spectrum disorders. *Am. J. Med.* 1984;77:812-22.

[21] Maricq HR, Harper FE, Khan MM, Tan EM, LeRoy EC. Microvascular abnormalities as possible predictors of disease subsets in Raynaud phenomenon and early connective tissue disease. *Clin. Exp. Rheumatol.* 1983;1:195-205.

[22] Andrade LE, Gabriel Júnior A, Assad RL, Ferrari AJ, Atra E. Panoramic nailfold capillaroscopy: a new reading method and normal range. *Semin. Arthritis Rheum.* 1990;20:21-31.

[23] Terreri MT, Andrade LE, Puccinelli ML, Hilário MO, Goldenberg J. Nail fold capillaroscopy: normal findings in children and adolescents. *Semin. Arthritis Rheum.* 1999;29:36-42.

[24] Herrick AL, Moore T, Hollis S, Jayson MI. The influence of age on nailfold capillary dimensions in childhood. *J. Rheumatol.* 2000;27:797-800.

[25] Merlen JF. Capillaroscopy at the nail bed in functioning people aged 70 and over. *Int. Angiol.* 1985;4(3):285-8.

[26] Grassi W, De Angelis R. Capillaroscopy: questions and answers. *Clin. Rheumatol.* 2007;26:2009-16.

[27] Bollinger A, Fagrell B. Collagen vascular disease and related disorders. In Bollinger A and Fagrell B (eds.) Clinical Capillaroscopy: a Guide to its Use in Clinical Research and Practice. Gottingen: Hogrefe and Huber Publishers 1990,pp. 121-143.

[28] Sulli A, Pizzorni C, Smith V, Zampogna G, Ravera F, Cutolo M. Timing of transition between capillaroscopic patterns in systemic sclerosis. *Arthritis Rheum.* 2012;64:821-5.

[29] Ingegnoli F, Zeni S, Gerloni V, Fantini F. Capillaroscopic observations in childhood rheumatic diseases and healthy controls. *Clin. Exp. Rheumatol.* 2005;23:905-11.

[30] Pavlov-Dolijanović S, Damjanov N, Ostojić P, Susić G, Stojanović R, Gacić D, Grdinić A. The prognostic value of nailfold capillary changes for the development of connective tissue disease in children and adolescents with primary raynaud phenomenon: a follow-up study of 250 patients. *Pediatr. Dermatol.* 2006;23:437-42.

[31] Navon P, Yarom A, Davis E. Raynaud's features in childhood. Clinical, immunological and capillaroscopic study. *J. Mal. Vasc.* 1992;17:273-6.

[32] Walker UA, Tyndall A, Czirják L, Denton C, Farge-Bancel D, Kowal-Bielecka O, et al. Clinical risk assessment of organ manifestations in

systemic sclerosis: a report from the EULAR Scleroderma Trials And Research group database. *Ann. Rheum. Dis.* 2007;66:754-63.

[33]   Fransen J, Johnson SR, van den Hoogen F, Baron M, Allanore Y, Carreira PE, et al. Items for developing revised classification criteria in systemic sclerosis: Results of a consensus exercise. *Arthritis Care Res.* (Hoboken) 2012;64:351-7.

[34]   Johnson SR, Fransen J, Khanna D, Baron M, van den Hoogen F, Medsger TA Jr, et al. Validation of potential classification criteria for systemic sclerosis. *Arthritis Care Res.* (Hoboken) 2012;64:358-67.

[35]   Pavlov-Dolijanovic S, Damjanov NS, Stojanovic RM, Vujasinovic Stupar NZ, Stanisavljevic DM. Scleroderma pattern of nailfold capillary changes as predictive value for the development of a connective tissue disease: a follow-up study of 3,029 patients with primary Raynaud's phenomenon. *Rheumatol. Int.* 2012;32:3039-45.

[36]   Cutolo M, Smith V, Sulli A. Training in capillaroscopy: a growing interest. *J. Rheumatol.* 2012;39:1113-6.

[37]   Weiner ES, Hildebrandt S, Senécal JL, Daniels L, Noell S, Joyal F,et al. Prognostic significance of anticentromere antibodies and anti-topoisomerase I antibodies in Raynaud's disease. A prospective study. *Arthritis Rheum.* 1991;34:68-77.

[38]   Hamaguchi Y. Autoantibody profiles in systemic sclerosis: predictive value for clinical evaluation and prognosis. *J. Dermatol.* 2010;37:42-53.

[39]   Schmidt KU, Mensing H. Are nailfold capillary changes indicators of organ involvement in progressive systemic sclerosis? *Dermatologica* 1988;176:18-21.

[40]   Cutolo M, Pizzorni C, Tuccio M, Burroni A, Craviotto C, Basso M, et al. Nailfold videocapillaroscopic patterns and serum autoantibodies in systemic sclerosis. *Rheumatology* (Oxford) 2004;43:719-26.

[41]   Koenig M, Joyal F, Fritzler MJ, Roussin A, Abrahamowicz M, Boire G, et al. Autoantibodies and microvascular damage are independent predictive factors for the progression of Raynaud's phenomenon to systemic sclerosis: a twenty-year prospective study of 586 patients, with validation of proposed criteria for early systemic sclerosis. *Arthritis Rheum.* 2008;58:3902-12.

[42]   Cutolo M, Sulli A, Pizzorni C, Smith V. Capillaroscopy as an Outcome Measure for Clinical Trials on the Peripheral Vasculopathy in SSc-Is It Useful? *Int. J. Rheumatol.* 2010;2010. pii: 784947. doi: 10.1155/2010/784947. Epub 2010 Aug 16.

[43] Valim V, Assis LS, Simões MF, Trevisani VF, Pucinelli ML, Andrade LE. Correlation between serum E-selectin levels and panoramic nailfold capillaroscopy in systemic sclerosis. *Braz. J. Med. Biol. Res.* 2004;37:1423-7.

[44] Del Rosso A, Distler O, Milia AF, Emanueli C, Ibba-Manneschi L, Guiducci S, Conforti ML, Generini S, Pignone A, Gay S, Madeddu P, Matucci-Cerinic M. Increased circulating levels of tissue kallikrein in systemic sclerosis correlate with microvascular involvement. *Ann. Rheum. Dis.* 2005 Mar;64(3):382-7.

[45] Sulli A, Soldano S, Pizzorni C, Montagna P, Secchi ME, Villaggio B, et al. Raynaud's phenomenon and plasma endothelin: correlations with capillaroscopic patterns in systemic sclerosis. *J. Rheumatol. 2009;36:1235*-9.

[46] Caramaschi P, Volpe A, Canestrini S, Bambara LM, Faccini G, Carletto A, Biasi D. Correlation between homocysteine plasma levels and nailfold videocapillaroscopic patterns in systemic sclerosis. *Clin. Rheumatol.* 2007;26:902-7.

[47] Mihai C, Tervaert JW. Anti-endothelial cell antibodies in systemic sclerosis. *Ann. Rheum. Dis.* 2010;69:319-24.

[48] Riccieri V, Germano V, Alessandri C, Vasile M, Ceccarelli F, Sciarra I, et al. More severe nailfold capillaroscopy findings and anti-endothelial cell antibodies. Are they useful tools for prognostic use in systemic sclerosis? *Clin. Exp. Rheumatol.* 2008;26:992-7.

[49] Volpe A, Biasi D, Caramaschi P, Mantovani W, Bambara LM, Canestrini S, et al. Levels of F2-isoprostanes in systemic sclerosis: correlation with clinical features. *Rheumatology* (Oxford) 2006;45:314-20.

[50] Caramaschi P, Canestrini S, Martinelli N, Volpe A, Pieropan S, Ferrari M, et al. Scleroderma patients nailfold videocapillaroscopic patterns are associated with disease subset and disease severity. *Rheumatology* (Oxford) 2007;46:1566-9.

[51] Smith V, Pizzorni C, De Keyser F, Decuman S, Van Praet JT, Deschepper E,et al. Reliability of the qualitative and semiquantitative nailfold videocapillaroscopy assessment in a systemic sclerosis cohort: a two-centre study. *Ann. Rheum. Dis.* 2010;69:1092-6.

[52] Alivernini S, De Santis M, Tolusso B, Mannocci A, Bosello SL, Peluso G, et al. Skin ulcers in systemic sclerosis: determinants of presence and predictive factors of healing. *J. Am. Acad. Dermatol.* 2009;60:426-35.

[53] Sebastiani M, Manfredi A, Vukatana G, Moscatelli S, Riato L, Bocci M, et al. Predictive role of capillaroscopic skin ulcer risk index in systemic sclerosis: a multicentre validation study. *Ann. Rheum. Dis.* 2012; 71:67-70.

[54] Bredemeier M, Xavier RM, Capobianco KG, Restelli VG, Rohde LE, Pinotti AF, et al. Nailfold capillary microscopy can suggest pulmonary disease activity in systemic sclerosis. *J. Rheumatol.* 2004;31:286-94.

[55] Hofstee HM, Vonk Noordegraaf A, Voskuyl AE, Dijkmans BA, Postmus PE, Smulders YM, Serné EH. Nailfold capillary density is associated with the presence and severity of pulmonary arterial hypertension in systemic sclerosis. *Ann. Rheum. Dis.* 2009;68:191-5.

[56] Ong YY, Nikoloutsopoulos T, Bond CP, Smith MD, Ahern MJ, Roberts-Thomson PJ. Decreased nailfold capillary density in limited scleroderma with pulmonary hypertension. *Asian Pac. J. Allergy Immunol.* 1998;16:81-6.

[57] Greidinger EL, Gaine SP, Wise RA, Boling C, Housten-Harris T, Wigley FM. Primary pulmonary hypertension is not associated with scleroderma-like changes in nailfold capillaries. *Chest* 2001;120:796-800.

[58] Cutolo M, Grassi W, Matucci Cerinic M. Raynaud's phenomenon and the role of capillaroscopy. *Arthritis Rheum.* 2003;48:3023-30.

[59] Jayson MI. The micro-circulation in systemic sclerosis. *Clin. Exp. Rheumatol.* 1984;2:85-91.

In: Scleroderma   ISBN: 978-1-62618-802-0
Editor: Romain De Winter   © 2013 Nova Science Publishers, Inc.

Chapter IV

Localized Scleroderma: Symptoms, Diagnosis and Treatment

Maria Teresa Garcia-Romero[1],
*Ronald Laxer[2] and Elena Pope[3],**

[1]Department of Pediatric Medicine, Dermatology Section
[2]Division of Rheumatology, Departments of Paediatrics and Medicine
[3]Department of Pediatric Medicine, Dermatology Section
The Hospital for Sick Children, University of Toronto, Toronto, Canada

Abstract

Scleroderma is a rare fibrosing disorder of the skin and underlying tissues characterized by skin thickening and hardening due to an increased collagen density. The approximate incidence varies according to race, but is approximately 0.4-2.7 per 100 000 persons. Its exact pathogenesis is still unknown, but several triggering factors in genetically predisposed individuals might lead to release of pro-inflammatory cytokines, which results in dysregulation of connective tissue metabolism

---

* Corresponding author: Elena Pope MD, MSc, FRCPC, Department of Pediatric Medicine, Dermatology Section, The Hospital for Sick Children, 555 University Avenue, Toronto, M5G 1X8 Canada. Phone: 416-813-8185; E-mail: elena.pope@sickkids.ca.

and ultimately to fibrosis. Scleroderma can be divided into localized scleroderma or morphea, which is the focus of this chapter, and systemic scleroderma (SSc). Several clinical forms of localized scleroderma exist including morphea en plaque, generalized morphea, guttate morphea, nodular morphea, subcutaneous morphea and linear scleroderma. Treatment depends on the type; circumscribed forms may benefit topical treatment, while generalized or linear lesions would require systemic treatment. Although localized scleroderma has a good prognosis in general, some clinical subtypes of the disease can be very deforming and irreversibly disabling, especially when affecting the extremities or the face.

Scleroderma (defined as "hard skin") describes a group of disorders in which the skin becomes progressively indurated and stiff as the end result of a complex interplay of immune, genetic and environmental factors. Scleroderma encompasses different conditions and has different clinical presentations. The most important distinction is whether scleroderma is localized (also known as morphea) or systemic (systemic scleroderma or sclerosis) (Table 1).

Localized scleroderma (LSc, also known as morphea) is a rare fibrosing disorder of the skin and underlying tissues. It is an inflammatory disorder characterized by skin thickening and hardening due to an increased collagen density. LSc can be differentiated from systemic sclerosis based on the appearance of the cutaneous manifestations and absence of severe internal organ involvement.

Table 1. Classification of scleroderma and related disorders

Systemic	Localized scleroderma or morphea	Others
Systemic sclerosis (SSc)	Circumscribed	Graft versus host disease
- Limited (lSSc)	Linear	(GVHD)
- Diffuse (dSSc)	Deep	Drug and toxin induced
Overlap diseases with	Pansclerotic	scleroderma
scleroderma	Mixed	Premature aging syndromes
-Mixed connective tissue		Phenylketonuria
disease		Scleromyxedema
-SSc - polymyositis		

Epidemiology

Epidemiologic studies have reported different incidence rates, up to 2.7 per 100 000 persons [1]. A female predominance of 2.4:1 has been reported. [2,3] Although morphea affects all races, it is more prevalent in Caucasians [1,2,3] This condition usually starts in childhood, especially the linear subtypes, with nearly 90% of children presenting between 2 and 14 years of age. There is another peak between 40 and 50 years of age for circumscribed or plaque morphea [4].

Etiology and Pathogenesis

The etiology and pathogenesis are not completely understood; current thinking points to a complex interplay of autoimmunity, environmental factors, and possibly infection and / or trauma triggering cytokine production and release responsible for increased fibroblast and collagen synthesis. Transforming growth factor (TGF) α and β, platelet-derived growth factor (PDGF), connective tissue growth factor (CTGF) and interleukin 4, 6 and 8, among others, have been shown to regulate fibroblast proliferation and extracellular matrix deposition as well as decrease matrix metalloproteinases (MMP), responsible for collagen degradation. [5] A family history of autoimmune conditions is present in 12% of cases; [2] however, in contrast to SSc, susceptibility genes for morphea have not been adequately studied. [5]. Among infectious agents, *Borrelia sp* organisms have been extensively studied, but their pathogenic role remains unclear. [5,4,6]

Clinical Presentations

Morphea is classified based on clinical presentations. Different classification schemes have been proposed, with the most clinically applicable including five morphea variants: circumscribed (with superficial and deep variants), generalized, linear (with trunk/limb variant and head variant), pansclerotic and mixed. (Table 2) [6] Other described variants such as guttate or bullous morphea are considered variants of these 5 subtypes, and other conditions such as atrophoderma of Pasini and Pierini, eosinophilic fascitis, lichen sclerosus et atrophicus are considered to be part of the spectrum of LSc. [1, 3, 7, 8, 9, 6, 2]

Table 2. Proposed classification of juvenile localized scleroderma

Main group	Subtype	Description
1. Circumscribed morphea	a. Superficial	Limited to dermis and epidermis. Single or multiple.
	b. Deep	Involves subcutaneous tissue, fascia, muscle. Single or multiple.
2. Linear scleroderma	a. Trunk, limbs	Linear induration involving dermis, subcutaneous tissue, muscle and bone.
	b. Head	En coup de sabre; Linear induration that affects face and scalp, may involve muscle and bone. Progressive hemifacial atrophy or Parry Romberg syndrome: Atrophy on one side of the face, mobile skin.
3. Generalized morphea		Four or more plaques larger than 3 cm that become confluent, involves at least 2 anatomic sites.
4. Pansclerotic morphea		Circumferential involvement of limbs or other areas of the body without internal organ involvement.
5. Mixed morphea		Combination of any of the previous subtypes.

Data from Laxer RM, Zulian F. Localized scleroderma. Curr Opin Rheumatol. 2006;18(6):606-13.

The most common presentation in children is linear morphea, either in extremities or on the head (en coup de sabre or Parry-Romberg syndrome / progressive hemifacial atrophy); and in adults it is circumscribed or plaque morphea. [6, 4]

Plaque or circumscribed morphea usually presents on the trunk, as an oval-shaped plaque, with a waxy, ivory sclerotic center, and an erythematous or violaceous (lilac ring) border. (Figure 1) It is confined to the dermis with occasional involvement of the subcutaneous fat tissue. Active lesions are often warm. Older lesions are atrophic, dyspigmented (hyper or hypopigmented), have varying degrees of sclerosis as well as loss of adnexal skin structures. There can be loss of dermal, subcutaneous and even muscular tissue depending on the depth.

Linear morphea is characterized by longitudinally arranged, band-like lesions located predominantly on the extremities, sometimes following the lines of Blaschko. [5] Deep involvement in a growing child may lead to localized growth retardation with a limb-length discrepancy, muscle atrophy (rarely myositis and myalgia), flexion contractures and significant disability. The "en coup de sabre" subtype of linear morphea occurs on the fronto-parietal region of the head, usually ranging from the hair-bearing scalp where it causes alopecia, to the forehead or even to the mandible. (Figure 2) Occasionally patients have involvement of the underlying central nervous system (CNS) manifested as headaches, seizures or ophthalmological findings such as uveitis or episcleritis. Some authors speculate that progressive facial hemiatrophy (Parry-Romberg syndrome) is a variant of linear morphea. This condition is characterized by primary atrophy of subcutaneous tissue, muscle and bone with little skin involvement. This often results in severe facial asymmetry. [5, 4, 6]

Figure 1. Plaque of active morphea with sclerotic, shiny ivory-like center and erythematous, lilac borders.

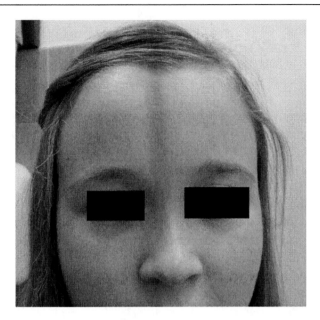

Figure 2. Patient with linear "en coup de sabre" morphea, there is an atrophic depressed hyperpigmented plaque going from the hair implantation line to the nose.

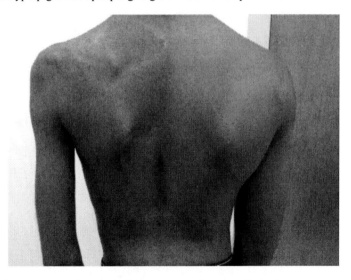

Figure 3. Patient with mixed morphea, there are circumscribed plaques on the trunk and linear deep morphea on the left arm. This patient also had linear deep involvement of the left lower extremity.

The deep type of morphea is extremely rare; the fibrotic process affects the deeper layers of connective tissue (fat, fascia and muscle) resulting in firm and bound down skin. It may manifest without any clinical signs of inflammation. [5, 4, 6]

Generalized morphea presents as four or more indurated plaques of more than 3 cm of diameter involving two or more anatomic sites. These can coalesce into larger lesions.

A rare variant of the generalized type is disabling pansclerotic morphea, which predominantly occurs in childhood, and leads to extensive involvement of the skin, fat, fascia, muscle and bone, resulting in severe contractures and disability. [5, 4, 6].

The mixed forms where different types of lesions are present simultaneously occur in 15% of patients. (Figure 3) [6]

Guttate morphea is a rare subtype that presents with multiple yellowish or whitish small sclerotic lesions with a shiny surface, primarily on the trunk. Atrophoderma of Pasini and Pierini is possibly an abortive type of morphea, where there is deeper atrophy and the lesions have a distinct cliff-border depression compared to the rest of the skin [4].

Eosinophilic fasciitis is considered by some authors to be a subtype of generalized morphea, which exclusively affects extremities and presents with a rapid onset of symmetrical swelling of the skin, progressively becoming indurated and fibrotic with a typical "peau d'orange-like" appearance [4].

Lichen sclerosus et atrophicus (LSA) is an condition in which patients develop very characteristic pale shiny atrophic plaques. It predominantly affects the anogenital area but it can present in any other part of the body. There is a high prevalence of LSA in patients with circumscribed and generalized morphea and it is also related to other autoimmune diseases, which is suggestive of a common pathogenic background. [10]

The natural course of a plaque of morphea includes various stages. Initially there is an early stage of inflammation including hyperemia and edema, followed by progressive fibrosis and sclerosis that has an ivory-appearance. Finally, there is an atrophic phase that leaves a dyspigmented atrophic plaque. This progression occurs over several years with variations from patient to patient and also depending on the subtype of morphea [1, 2, 3, 7, 8].

Approximately 40% of children with morphea have extracutaneous manifestations such as arthritis, neurologic symptoms (headache, seizures), vascular abnormalities (Raynaud phenomenon), ocular involvement, gastrointestinal and respiratory symptoms [4, 3, 11]. In linear scleroderma involving the face, neurological involvement such as seizures or brain calcifications and ocular changes like uveitis or episcleritis have also been described. [4, 5]

Patients with morphea very frequently have positive antinuclear antibodies (ANA)(23 to 73%); [6, 5] less commonly positive anti-histone antibodies (AHA) and anti-single stranded DNA (ssDNA) serology may be seen in up to 34%, but these antibodies are not associated with disease activity and are of limited clinical utility. [12] In a recent study, 46% adult patients and 12.6% pediatric patients with morphea were found to have anticardiolipin antibodies. [13] Patients with active morphea may also present positive rheumatoid factor [6] hypergammaglobulinemia and eosinophilia. [5] Elevation of various cytokines and chemokines, including tumor necrosis factor (TNF) α and interleukin (IL)-13 has been reported [14]

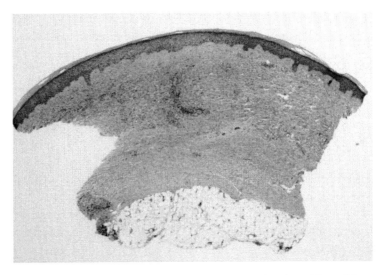

Figure 4. Histological features of morphea, there is excessive deposition of dense collagen from the dermis to the subcutaneous fat with a perivascular and periadnexal lymphohystiocytic inflammatory infiltrate. The eccrine glands become atrophied as the hypertrophied collage surrounds them and the subcutaneous fat appears "trapped" in the dermis because of the extension of collagen into the subcutaneous tissues.

Typically, clinical activity in morphea persists for 3 to 4 years, but new lesions can develop even after longer periods. At the most severe spectrum of the disease, patients may have growth retardation, irreversible structural deformities, joint contractures and severe disabilities: functional, cosmetic or psychological. Even if the condition undergoes remission, the residual damage created by active disease (pigment change, atrophy, contracture, limb length discrepancy) may be severe. [15]

Diagnosis

The diagnosis of morphea is mainly clinical; however, its rarity combined with stage dependent clinical presentation may result in misdiagnosis in early stages. Studies have shown significant delay in many cases, from 6 months up to years. [12, 16, 17]

The diagnosis can be made through history and careful examination of the skin. The appearance of lesions changes over time, so asking patients about the clinical evolution is helpful, as is a review of early photographs that the family may have. Patients often present with multiple lesions in different stages of evolution. The diagnosis is also aided by finding specific patterns of morphology: plaque, linear, generalized, guttate, superficial or deep.

A biopsy is sometimes necessary to confirm the diagnosis. Histologically, early inflammatory stages are characterized by a mixed perivascular infiltrate of predominantly lymphocytes with rare plasma cells and eosinophils in the reticular dermis. In the later stages there is excessive deposition of dense collagen. The eccrine glands become atrophied as the hypertrophied collage surrounds them and the subcutaneous fat appears "trapped" in the dermis because of the extension of collagen into the subcutaneous tissues. (Figure 4) Lichen sclerosus et atrophicus' characteristic histological findings are an atrophic epidermis and edematous homogenized hyalinized collagen in the papillary dermis.

These changes can be found in combination with deeper alterations when the plaques or morphea are both superficial and deep. Calcification, myositis, myofibrosis and bone atrophy may also occur [1, 3, 2, 7].

Differential Diagnoses

- Lipodermatosclerosis
- Trauma-induced fat necrosis
- Chronic graft-versus-host disease
- Nephrogenic systemic fibrosis
- Pretibial myxedema

- Connective tissue nevi
- Morpheaform basal cell carcinoma
- Lyme disease (acrodermatitis chronica atrophicans)
- Vitiligo
- Cutaneous T-cell lymphoma
- Scleromyxedemal Dermatofibrosarcoma protuberans
- Lupus erythematous profundus
- Other panniculitis
- Porphyria cutanea tarda
- Focal dermal hypoplasia
- Fibromatosis

Other Diagnostic and Assessment Tools

Detection of disease activity remains a fundamental challenge, both for evaluating the need for treatment and assessment of therapeutic efficacy over time. Indicators of disease activity include development of new lesions, extension of existing lesions, erythema and/or induration of the advancing edge, patient-reported symptoms such as tingling. Disease damage manifests as pigmentary changes, induration of the center, atrophy at any level, contracture, limb-length discrepancy and scarring alopecia. Facial deformities can be significant. Reliable and reproducible methods are needed to detect and monitor disease activity, since it is at this stage that lesions can be treated and damage prevented.

Several clinical scales have been developed in the last few years to assess disease activity, such as the validated localized scleroderma skin severity index (LoSSI) which measures skin erythema, thickness and new lesions in each of 18 anatomic areas. The localized scleroderma skin damage index (LoSDI) measures disease damage. Currently, it is recommended to combine both indexes in a composite score: localized scleroderma cutaneous assessment tool (LoSCAT) [19, 20].

The DIET scale is another proposed way of evaluating a plaque of morphea according to dyspigmentation (D), induration (I), erythema (E) and telangiectasias (T). This validated tool is of limited value outside the realm of research [21].

Thermography is a noninvasive technique that detects infrared radiation. It has been previously reported as having a very high sensitivity and specificity as a marker of activity in morphea. [22, 23]

Other methods of measuring disease activity have been reported, such as devices to evaluate skin thickness (plicometer [24] or durometer[25, 26] laser Doppler flowmetry, [27, 28] ultrasound, [29, 30] magnetic resonance imaging [8] and a computerized method [31] to assess induration and surface area.

Management

The management of severe localized scleroderma is challenging. The choice of treatment will depend on the extent, location, depth and progression of the condition. For patients with localized plaques of morphea without any restriction in movement or growth or development, topical treatment is an excellent option. There are many options available such as topical corticosteroids and vitamin D3 analogues such as calcipotriene, which have been used traditionally. Imiquimod is an immunomodulator which upregulates interferon α and γ and inhibits the collagen production by fibroblasts likely by downregulating TGF-β, it is particularly effective in more indurated lesions. [32] Topical tacrolimus has also been found to improve localized plaques. [33] Local phototherapy with ultraviolet A1 radiation (UVA1), with or without psoralen, and narrow band ultraviolet B (NB UVB) is another possible choice, especially for superficial lesions, but true evidence of efficacy is lacking particularly in the paediatric population. [7, 33, 9, 34, 21, 15, 6, 5, 35]

In general terms, morphea lesions that have potential of causing functional or cosmetic disfigurement should be treated systemically. These include linear lesions of the extremity crossing over a joint, linear lesions on the face or generalized forms. [5, 7, 36, 9]

The combination of low-dose methotrexate (MTX) and systemic corticosteroids (CS), either given as pulses with intravenous (IV) methylprednisolone or oral prednisone, has shown very good response rates and excellent tolerability. [36, 35, 37, 38] Other treatments that have been used with variable success rates are phototherapy, antimalarials, IV immuno-globulin, interpheron gamma, D-penicillamine, cyclosporine, tacrolimus, mycophenolate mofetil (MMF) [38] and imatinib. [1, 2, 7, 33, 15, 5, 6]

Table 3. Algorithm for the management of localized scleroderma

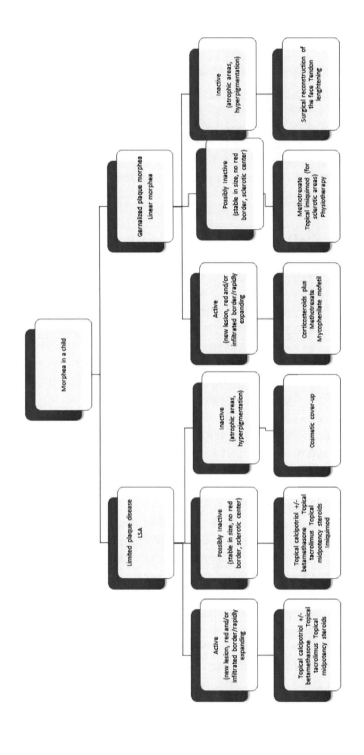

Although there is some evidence on the effectiveness of systemic intervention, the ideal combination, dosage and duration is currently not known.

Current recommendations from the CARRA group of investigators studying clinical effectiveness protocols are that moderately or highly severe localized scleroderma be treated systemically for the initial 12 months either with MTX alone, MTX plus CS (IV methylprednisolone or oral prednisone) or MMF for patients who did not tolerate or did not respond to treatment with MTX. The accorded dose of methotrexate was 1 mg/kg/week, preferently SC (maximum 25 mg/kg/week); of IV methylprednisolone 30 mg/kg/dose IV (max 1 gr) for 3 consecutive days/month for 3 months or 1 dose/week for 12 weeks; of prednisone 2 mg/kg/day PO (max 60mg) twice a day for 2-4 weeks followed by a tapering schedule; and of MMF 600 to 1000 mg twice a day according to weight [39].

As previously stated, assessment of disease activity or progression is key in choosing the best therapeutic option. Systemic treatment should be continued for at least one year after the disease is deemed to be inactive. Even then, the impact of therapy on long-term disease outcomes is not clear, as there is a moderately high recurrence rate of disease activity after discontinuation of therapy, ranging from 15.4% up to 28%, especially in patients with the linear limb subtype and older age of onset [17, 37]

Once the disease is inactive without treatment for at least 2 years and the pediatric patient has reached full growth, damage can be addressed and treated depending on the impairment caused. If it is functional, patients should be assessed for orthotics or orthopedics, oral maxillofacial or plastic surgery; if the impairment is cosmetic, injectable fillers or autologous fat transplantation can be contemplated with very good outcomes and patient satisfaction rates. (Table 3) [15, 40]

Prognosis

Overall, the prognosis of morphea in plaques is good. The linear and deep subtypes can have severe resultant morbidity, both cosmetic and functional.

References

[1]   Peterson LS, Nelson AM, Su WP, Mason T, O'Fallom WM et al. The epidemiology of morphea (localized scleroderma) in Olmsted County 1960-1993. *J Rheumatol.* 1997; 24:73-80.

[2]   Zulian F, Athreya BH, Laxer R, Nelson AM, Feitosa de Oliveria SK, Punaro G, et al. Juvenile localized scleroderma: clinical and epidemiological features in 750 children. An international study. *Rheumatol.* 2006 ;45: 614-620.

[3]   Christen-Zaech S, Hakim MD, Afsar FS, Paller AS. Pediatric morphea (localized scleroderma): Review of 136 patients. *J Am Acad Dermatol.*2008: 59:385-96.

[4]   Atzeni F, Bardoni A, Cutolo M et al. Localized and systemic forms of scleroderma in adults and children. *Clin Exp Rheumatol.* 2006;24(suppl.40):S36-45.

[5]   Kreuter A. Localized scleroderma. *Dermatol Ther.* 2012;25:135-147.

[6]   Laxer RM, Zulian F. Localized scleroderma. *Curr Opin Rheumatol.* 2006;18:606-13.

[7]   Murray KJ, Laxer RM. Scleroderma in children and adolescents. *Rheum Dis Clin N Am.* 2002;28:603-624.

[8]   Fett N, Werth VP. Update on Morphea: Part I. Epidemiology, clinical presentation and pathogenesis. *J Am Acad Dermatol.* 2011;64(2):217-28.

[9]   Uziel Y, Krafchik BR, Silverman ED, Thorner PS, Laxer RM. Localized scleroderma in childhood: a report of 30 cases. *Semin Arthritis Rheum.* 1994; 23:328-40.

[10]   Kreuter A, Wischnewski J, Terras S, Altmeyer P, Stuckeer M et al. Coexistence of lichen sclerosus and morphea: a retrospective analysis of 472 patients with localized scleroderma from a German tertiary referral center. *J Am Acad Dermatol.* 2012;67:1157-62.

[11]   Zulian F, Vallongo C, Woo P, Russo R, Ruperto N, Harper J, et al. Localized scleroderma in childhood is not just a skin disease. *Arthritis Rheum.* 2005;52:2873-81.

[12]   Nouri S, Jacobe H. Recent developments in diagnosis and assessment of morphea. *Curr Rheumatol Rep.* 2013;15:308.

[13] Sato S, Fujimoto M, Hasegawa M, Takehara K. Antiphospholipid antibody in localised scleroderma. *Ann Rheum Dis.* 2003;62:771–774.

[14] Hasegawa M, Sato S, Nagaoka T, et al. Serum levels of tumor necrosis factor and interleukin-13 are elevated in patients with localized scleroderma. *Dermatol.* 2003;207:141–147.

[15] Zwischenberger BA, Jacobe HT. A systematic review of morphea treatments and therapeutic algorithm. *J Am Acad Dermatol.* 2011;65:925-41.

[16] Johnson W, Jacobe H. Morphea in adults and children cohort II: patients with morphea experience delay in diagnosis and large variation in treatment. *J Am Acad Dermatol.* 2012;67:881-9.

[17] Mirsky L, Chakkittakandiyil A, Laxer R, O'Brien C, Pope E. Relapse after systemic treatment in pediatric morphea. *Br J Dermatol.* 2012;166:443-5.

[18] Succaria F, Kurban M, Kibbi AG, Abbas O. Clinicopathological study of 81 cases of localized and systemic scleroderma. *JEADV* 2013; 27:e191-6.

[19] Arkachaisri T, Vilaiyuk S, Torok KS, Medsger TA. Development and initial validation of the Localized Scleroderma Skin Damage Index and Physician Global Assessment of disease Damage: a proof-of-concept study. *Rheumatol.* 2010;49:373-381.

[20] Arkachaisri T, Vilaiyuk S, Li S, O'Neil KM, Pope E, Higgins GC et al. The Localized Scleroderma Skin Severity Index and Physician Global Assessment of disease Activity: A work in progress toward development of localized scleroderma outcome measures. *J Rheumatol.* 2009;36:2819-29.

[21] Cunningham BB, Landells ID, Langman C, Sailer DE, Paller AS. Topical calcipotriene for morphea/linear scleroderma. J Am Acad Dermatol. 1998;39:211-5.

[22] Martini G, Murray KJ, Howell KJ, Harper J, Atherton D, Woo P et al. Juvenile-onset localized scleroderma activity detection by infrared thermography. *Rheumatology* (Oxford) 2002;41:1178-82.

[23] Birdi N, Shore A, Rush P, Laxer RM, Silverman ED, Krafchik B. Childhood linear scleroderma: a possible role of thermography for evaluation. *J Rheumatol.* 1992;19:968-73.

[24] . Nives PM, Castagneto C, Filaci G, Murdaca G, Puppo F, Indiveri F et al. Plicometer skin test: a new technique for the evaluation of cutaneous involvement in systemic sclerosis. *Br J Rheumatol.* 1997;36:244-50.

[25] Seyger MM, van den Hoogen FH, de Boo T, de Jong EM. Reliability of two methods to assess morphea: skin scoring and the use of a durometer. *J Am Acad Dermatol* 1997;37:793-6.

[26] Falanga V, Bucalo B. Use of a durometer to assess skin hardness. *J Am Acad Dermatol* 1993;29:47-51.

[27] Weibel L, Howell KJ, Visentin MT, Rudiger A, Denton CP, Zulian F et al. Laser Doppler flowmetry for assessing localized scleroderma in children. *Arthritis and Rheumatism* 2007;56(10):3489-95.

[28] Moore TL, Vij S, Murray AK, Bhushan M, Griffiths CE, Herrick AL. Pilot study of dual-wavelength (532 and 633 nm) laser Doppler imaging and infrared thermography of morphoea. *Br J Dermatol.* 2009;160(4):864-7.

[29] Cosnes A, Anglade MC, Revuz J, Radier C. Thirteen-megahertz ultrasound probe: its role in diagnosing localized scleroderma. *Br J Dermatol* 2003;148:724-9.

[30] Szymanska E, Nowicki A, Mlosek K, Litniewski J, Lewandowski M, Secomski W et al. Skin imaging with high frequency ultrasound - preliminary results. *Eur J Ultrasound* 2000;12:9-16.

[31] Zulian F, Meneghesso D, Grisan E, Vittadello F, Belloni Fortina A, Pigozzi B et al. A new computerized method for the assessment of skin lesions in localized scleroderma. *Rheumatol* 2007;46:856-860.

[32] Zulian F, Laxer RM. Localized sclerodermas. In: Cassidy JT, Petty RE, Laxer RM, Lindsley CB. *Textbook of Pediatric Rheumatology.* Philadelphia : Saunders Elsevier, 2011.

[33] Fett N, Werth VP. Update on Morphea: Part II. *J Am Acad Dermatol* 2011;64:231-42.

[34] Gupta AK, Browne M, Bluhm R. Imiquimod: a review. *J Cutan Med Surg* 2002;6:554-60.

[35] Sapadin AN, Fleischmajer R. Treatment of scleroderma. *Arch Dermatol* 2002;138:99-105.

[36] Uziel Y, Feldman BM, Krafchik BR, Yeung RS, Laxer RM. Methotrexate and corticosteroid therapy for pediatric localized scleroderma. *J Pediatr* 2000;136:91-5.

[37] Zulian F, Vallongo C, Patrizi A et al. Long-term follow-up study of methotrexate in juvenile localized scleroderma (morphea). *J Am Acad Dermatol* 2012;67:151-6.

[38] Martini G, Ramanan AV, Falcini F, Girschick H, Goldsmith DP, Zulian F. Successful treatment of severe or methotrexate-resistant juvenile localized scleroderma with mycophenolate mofetil. *Rheumatology* 2009; 48: 1410–3.

[39] Li SC, Torok KS, Pope E, Dedeoglu F, Hong S, Jacobe HT et al. Development of consensus treatment plans for juvenile localized scleroderma: a roadmap toward comparative effectiveness studies in juvenile localized scleroderma. *Arthritis Care Res* 2012;64(8):1175-85.

[40] Palmero ML, Uziel Y, Laxer RM, Forrest CR, Pope E. En coup de sabre scleroderma and Parry-Romberg syndrome in adolescents: surgical options and patient related outcomes. *J Rheumatol* 2010;37:2174-9.

In: Scleroderma
Editor: Romain De Winter

ISBN: 978-1-62618-802-0
© 2013 Nova Science Publishers, Inc.

Chapter V

Evaluation of a New CENPB Epitope Array for Systemic Sclerosis-Associated Centromere Autoantibodies

Iván Rodríguez[1], Khaoula Hamdouch[1],
Carmen Rodríguez[2], Jose Perez-Venegas[3],
Mohcine Bennani[4], Manuela Ortiz[1]
and Manuel M. Valdivia[1]

[1]Departamento de Biomedicina Biotecnología y Salud Publica,
Facultad de Ciencias, Universidad de Cádiz, Puerto Real, Cádiz, Spain
[2]Servicio de Inmunología, Hospital Puerta del Mar, Cádiz, Spain,
[3]Servicio de Reumatología, Hospital General de Jerez,
Jerez de la Frontera, Cádiz, Spain
[4]Equipe de Génomique Humaine, Ziaten, Tanger, Maroc

Abstract

Systemic sclerosis (SSc) is a heterogeneous autoimmune disorder characterized by the presence of antinuclear autoantibodies (ANA). The ANA classically detected in SSc include anticentromere antibodies

(ACA) which are positive in 50-60% of the patients. The centromere protein CENPB is a major autoantigen reactive with SSc sera showing a typical immunofluorescence staining pattern. Previously, epitopes on CENPB were identified in the N-terminal (Nt) and C-terminal (Ct) domains of the autoantigen and this form the rationale for an specific multi-parallel detection of CENPB epitopes in SSc. Using recombinant CENPB Nt and Ct domains we have developed a new fluorescent array immunoassay for ACA detection in SSc patients. 81 sera from patients with SSc, SLE and normal controls were evaluated. From 27 ACA positive sera tested, 25 were CENPB positive by ECL blot techniques. Among them our fluorescent array showed 23 Nt-CENPB and 12 Ct-CENPB positives. 10 Ct-CENPB were also Nt-CENPB positive by the array assay. 13 Nt-CENPB were Ct-CENPB negative and only 2 Ct-CENPB positive sera were Nt-CENPB negative. This result shows a prevalence of Nt-CENPB epitope over Ct-CENPB in ACA positive SSc patients. The CENPB fluorescent array developed has good agreement with conventional techniques for selected ACA and has the advantage of multi-parallel detection of CENPB autoepitopes in SSc.

Introduction

Autoantibodies against specific cell components are often the serological hallmark of autoimmune diseases. Among them nuclear components are the targets of selective autoimmune response in certain patients with rheumatic diseases. Thus, scleroderma is characterized by ANA which are useful for diagnosis of this heterogeneous disease. Other autoantibodies are also detected in SSc but they are associated in varying degree of clinical significance. Five major autoantibodies named, anticentromere, anti-topoI, anti-RNA polymerase III anti Th/To and anti-fibrillarin account for 75-80% of ANAs in SSc [1]. Among these, anti-centromere antibodies are useful biomarkers in the diagnosis of SSc. ACA are found in 20% to 40% of SSc patients, and detection of these autoantibodies is done primarily by IF on Hep-2 human cells and interpretation of the immunostaining pattern is a straight forward step. Although ACA were initially observed in limited sclerosis or CREST Syndrome [2,3], they have also been detected in other rheumatic diseases including Sjögren's syndrome [4-6].

ACA usually bind at least one of three major centromere proteins named as CENPA, CENPB and CENPC [7]. Studies of sera from SSc patients with anti-centromere immunofluorescence positive pattern showed that 93.5% were found to have anti-CENPA reactivity and 95.4% anti-CENPB reactivity by

ELISA [8]. Traditionally CENPB (80 kDa) was thought to be the major antigen reactive with SSc sera [2]. However, by ELISA analysis it was later found that antibodies to the N-terminal domain of CENPA were a more specific and earlier diagnostic marker of SSc than anti-CENPB [9]. In general, IF, ELISA and blots tests for CENPA and CENPB, yield results with similar sensitivity and specificity for the diagnosis of SSc [10]. In this regard, a blot assay with purified recombinant CENPB is currently used in clinical diagnosis of SSc (Innogenetics N.V.).

Person to person variability of a drug response is a significant problem in clinical practice and in drug development in autoimmune diseases. Recently, protein microarrays arise as a powerful technology which allows the simultaneous screening of a variety of antigens [11]. A recent multi-parallel line immunoassay for systemic sclerosis-associated autoantibodies was described to be in good agreement with other conventional techniques and good diagnostic utility [12]. Furthermore, the identification of specific epitopes in human autoantigens could provide insights on the disease pathogenicity mechanism. Many reports form the rationale for testing centromere autoantigens separately and not relying on IF alone [13]. In this regard, we developed a novel fluorescent array assay to investigate the contribution of CENPB domains to the antigenicity of centromere response in a group of SSc autoimmune patients.

Material and Methods

Human CENPB cDNAs were subcloned as Nt (1-350 aa) and Ct (540-599 aa) in pET11 and pET15b vectors and expressed in BL21 DE3 *E.coli* cells. Briefly, overnight cultures of transformed *E. coli* cells were diluted 1:50 in fresh L-Broth media containing ampicillin and grow for 2-3 hours at 37°C until 0.6 absorbance was reached. Then, IPTG was added to a final concentration of 1.0 mM and the cultures were grown at 30°C for 12-16 hours. Cells were pelleted and resuspended in PBS containing 1 mM of a protease inhibitor cocktail (Hoffmann-La Roche). Then, the cells were lysed by sonication on ice three times for 1 min each and centrifuged at 10000 rpm for 30 min at 4°C. The pellet of inclusion bodies were resuspended in 8M urea solution in PBS, diluted to 4M urea and used in SDS PAGE for further purification to homogeneity of Nt and Ct CENPB protein bands used in the array assay. Purified recombinant CENPB fragments were further analyzed by

SDS-PAGE and proved for specificity by western blot analysis with monospecific anti CENPB peptide antibodies made against the Nt and Ct terminal domains of CENPB antigen (data not shown).

Human autoimmune sera were obtained from the Immunology Service of Hospital Puerta del Mar, Cadiz, Spain, and used according to the rules and with the approval of the local ethics committees and the institutional review board. SSc patients were initially selected based on centromere positive pattern by immunofluorescence. Secondly SSc sera were also tested for CENPB positive reaction by western blots, done by a commercial blot assay (Innogenetics N.V.) (data not shown).

Arrays for Nt and Ct domains of CENPB were generated by spotting the recombinant proteins Nt (250 ng/μl and Ct (280 ng/μl) in 4M urea on nitrocellulose coated FAST slides (Whatman, GE Healthcare) using the MicroCaster manual microarraying system (Schleicher & Schuell). Several spots of buffer alone, BSA or recombinant Nt CENPI were also printed as negative controls for putative non-specific signals in the CENPB array. Approximately 20 to 70 nl of liquid was deposited per spot (spot diameter 500 to 1000 μm). Differences in size of the spot were probably due to the use of urea buffer to dissolve the arrayed protein and also intrinsic to the manual spotting used (MicroCaster system). After printing, samples on the slides were UV crosslinked, blocked with 3% BSA in PBS (blocking buffer) for at least 1 hour and left in a humid chamber until use. The slides were stables for several weeks when stored at 4°C. For antibody assay, the slides were rewashed with PBS-0.1% Tween (washing buffer) for 5-10 min. and mounted into a FAST Frame adapter with 16-pad incubation chambers (Whatman, GE Healthcare). Then, they were incubated at 37°C for 45 min with specific (Nt or Ct) anti-CENPB rabbit sera at proper dilution in blocking buffer. The slides were then washed with washing buffer three times for 10 min each, and incubated for 1 hour with biotin conjugated anti-rabbit IgG diluted 1: 4000 in blocking buffer. The slides were washed at room temperature three times of 10 min each with PBS-Tween and incubated for 1 hour with Cy3 labeled streptavidin PA 4300 diluted 1:6000 (Amersham Biosciences). Then the slides were washed 3 times with washing buffer for 10 min each, once with PBS and stored in PBS at 4°C until dried for scanning analysis. A similar experimental protocol was used to develop a CENPB array for analysis of human SSc centromere sera. In these cases human sera were assayed at 1:100 dilution and biotin labeled anti-human IgG and Cy3 labeled streptavidin were used. For each array, optimal concentration of antigens, dilutions of sera and conjugated antibodies were established after routine control titration experiments.

Analyses of the arrays were performed with a GenePix 4100A Microarray Scanner at 532 nm for Cy3. Bit images were generated with GenePix Pro 6.0 software (Axon Instruments, Molecular Devices Corp). The fluorescence intensity of each spot was measured and signal to local-background ratios were calculate by using the background subtraction of the GenePix Pro and deviations from the expected spot position were considered using the corresponding setting. The array results were considered positive when signal intensities exceeded those of the negative controls by applying the CPI (Composite Pixel Intensity) factor of the GenePix Pro software.

Results and Discussion

To study major CENPB epitopes recognized by ACA from SSc patients, we first developed a specific CENPB array assay by using recombinant proteins and monospecific anti-CENPB sera to the Nt and Ct CENPB domains. It should be noted that the expression level of particular domains of CENPB as fusion protein in *E.coli* is much higher than that of the whole CENPB protein, whereas its antigenicity appeared to be as high as that of the longer CENPB protein [14]. Thus, the high expression level of linear Nt and Ct CENPB fragments in *E. coli* cultures allows a straight forward purification of relatively large amounts of recombinant proteins. This material is very suitable as antigen source for an array system for routine screening of anti CENPB epitope autoantibodies. Results of our array analysis of Nt and Ct CENPB domains with monospecific anti-CENPB antibodies is shown in figure 1. As shown in figure 1(A, B), antigen and serum dilutions correlate well with the intensity of the spot signal observed. In each case it was a high correlation among signal intensities above background. A quality control of the spotting procedure and reproducibility of the array was performed by including four replicates of the same antigen in each square of the nitrocellulose slide. Similar results were obtained in parallel using an array for the Nt-CENPI human centromeric protein with a monospecific anti-CENPI serum (figure 1C). When mixed antigens, Nt-CENPB, Ct-CENPB and Nt-CENPI, were analyzed in a multiplexed array with different specific antibodies, the specificity of each array was demonstrated (figure 1D).

We applied the developed CENPB array to analyze SSc sera from patients harboring anticentromere CENPB reactivity. These sera were tested previously by western blots against full-length recombinant protein (data not shown). The specificity and sensitivity of the array was validated in our assay for identification of CENPB epitope domains. We assayed by the array 25 CENPB blot positive sera from SSc patients. In our analysis 23 sera showed Nt-CENPB reactivity and 12 were Ct-CENPB positive. In figure 2A-D examples of those array results are shown for both CENPB domains. These analyses corroborated well with those obtained by western blots (data not shown) and were demonstrated to be an alternative for the analysis of specific CENPB epitopes in human anticentromere response in SSc. In our report, although the number of sera studied was small, we found clearly that the Nt region of CENPB (1-350 aa) harbors more reactivity as an autoimmune epitope than the C-terminal domain tested (535-595 aa).

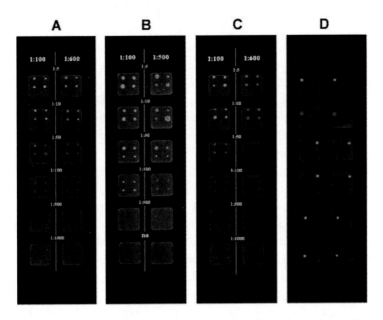

Figure 1. Develop of a specific array for Nt and Ct CENPB antigens. Recombinant antigens, Nt-CENPB in A, and Ct-CENPB in B, were spotted in quadruplicated in each nitrocellulose square. Recombinant Nt-CENPI antigen was used instead in C. Monospecific antibodies were used against Nt-CENPB (A), Ct-CENPB (B) and Nt-CENPI (C). Antigen and antibody dilutions are indicated in the figure. Specificity of the array is shown in D when mixed antigens were spotted in each nitrocellulose square; Nt CENPB was in left upper level, Ct CENPB in right upper level, Nt CENPI in left low level and BSA in right lower level in each nitrocellulose square. Groups of nitrocellulose square were developed with monospecific anti-Nt CENPB antibody (four upper ones), anti-Ct CENPB serum (four middle ones) and anti-CENPI antibody (four lower ones).

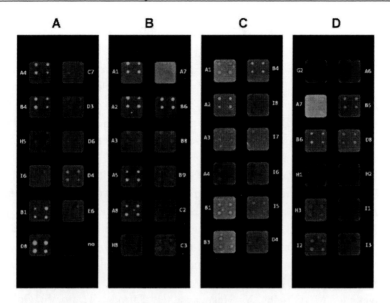

Figure 2. Analysis of human CENPB autoimmune sera by epitope array. Examples of reactivity of human SSc anti centromere sera against Nt CENPB (A and B) and Ct CENPB (C and D) antigens is shown. Letters and numbers mean different patients. Absence of antigen spotted in the array is indicating by no.

Conclusion

The CENPB protein array that was developed served to identify specific linear epitopes on the centromeric autoantigen. Interestingly, our results showed a clear predominance of Nt CENPB epitope over the Ct CENPB domain in SSc patients with anti centromere autoimmune response. This finding could give some insights into the pathogenetic mechanisms involved in the anticentromere response in human patients.

It remains to be evaluated using a larger sample size whether anti-CENPB detected by epitope specific assay such as the reported here, would have additional diagnostic value compared with whole CENPB blot. The application of a similar approach using arrays covering other centromere autoantigen such as CENPA, CENPC and others [15, 16] could provide a more specific diagnosis of the immune response in SSc disease.

References

[1]   Koening, M; Dieude, M; Senecal, JL. Predictive value of antinuclear autoantibodies: the lessons of the systemic sclerosis autoantibodies. *Autoimmun Rheum*, 2008, 7, 588-593.

[2]   Earnshaw, W; Bordwell, B; Marino, C; Rothfield, N. Three human chromosomal autoantigens are recognized by sera from patients with anti-centromere antibodies. *J Clin Invest.* 1986, 77(2), 426-430.

[3]   Tan, EM; Rodnan, GP; Garcia, I; Moroi, Y; Fritzler, MJ; Peebles, C. Diversity of antinuclear antibodies in progressive systemic sclerosis. Anticentromere antibody and its relationship to CREST syndrome. *Arthr Rheum*, 1980, 23, 617-625.

[4]   Muro, YJ; Sugimoto, K; Okazaki, T; Ohashi, M. The heterogeneity of anticentromere antibodies in immunoblotting analysis. *J. Rheumatol*, 1990, 17, 1042-1047.

[5]   Nakano, M; Ohuchi, Y; Hasegawa, H; Kuroda, T; Ito, S; Gejyo, F. Clinical significance of anticentromere antibodies in patients with systemic lupus erythematosus, *J Rheumatol.* 2000, 27(6), 1403-1407.

[6]   Gelber, AC; Pillemer, SR; Baum, BJ; Wigley, FM; Hummers, LK; Morris, S; Rosen, A; Casciola-Rosen, L. Distinct recognition of antibodies to centromere proteins in primary Sjogren's syndrome compared with limited scleroderma. *Ann Rheum Dis.* 2006, 65(8), 1028-1032.

[7]   Onozuka, Y; Shibata. M; Yonezawa, H; Terauti, K; Miyachi, K; Ueno, Y. Clinical significance of anticentromere antibody and anti-CENP-B antibody in sera of patients with primary biliary cirrhosis. *Rinsho Byori.* 1996, 44(9), 877-882.

[8]   Vázquez-Abad, D; Grodzicky, T; Senécal, JL. Anticentromere autoantibodies in patients without Raynaud's disease or systemic sclerosis. *Clin Immunol.* 1999, 90(2), 182-189.

[9]   Mahler, M; Maes, L; Blockmans, D; Westhovens, R; Bossuyt, X; Riemekasten, G; Schneider; S; Hiepe, F; Swart, A; Gürtler, I; Egerer, K; Fooke, M; Fritzler, MJ. Clinical and serological evaluation of a novel CENP-A peptide based ELISA. *Arthr Res Ther.* 2010, 12(3), R99.

[10]   Russo, K; Hoch, S; Dima, C; Varga, J; Teodorescu, M. Circulating anticentromere CENP-A and CENP-B antibodies in patients with diffuse and limited systemic sclerosis, systemic lupus erythematosus, and rheumatoid arthritis. *J Rheumatol.* 2000, 27(1), 142-148.

[11] Robinson, WH; DiGennaro, C; Hueber, W; Haab, BB; Kamachi, M; Dean, EJ; Fournel, S; Fong, D; Genovese, MC; de Vegvar, HE; Skriner. K; Hirschberg, DL; Morris, RI; Muller, S; Pruijn. GJ; van Venrooij, WJ; Smolen, JS; Brown, PO; Steinman, L; Utz, PJ. Autoantigen microarrays for multiplex characterization of autoantibody responses. *Nat Med.* 2002, 8(3), 295-301.

[12] Low, AHL; Wong, S; Thumboo, J; Hg, SC; Lim, JY; Ng, X; Earnest, A; Fong, KY. Evaluation of a new multi-parallel line immunoassay for systemic sclerosis-associated antibodies in an Asian population. *Rheumatology*, 2012, 51(8), 1465-1470.

[13] Mahler, M; Mierau, R; Genth, E; Blüthner, M. Development of a CENP-A/CENP-B-specific immune response in a patient with systemic sclerosis. *Arthritis Rheum.* 2002, 46(7), 1866-1872.

[14] Verheijen, R; de Jong, BA; Oberyé, EH; van Venrooij, WJ. Molecular cloning of a major CENP-B epitope and its use for the detection of anticentromere autoantibodies. *Mol Biol Rep.* 1992, 16(1), 49-59. .

[15] Song, G; Hu, C; Zhu, H; Wang, L; Zhang. F; Li, Y; Wu, L. New Centromere Autoantigens identified in systemic sclerosis using centromere protein microarrays. *J Rheumatol*, 2013, Feb 15.

[16] Hamdouch, K; Rodríguez, C; Perez-Venegas, J; Rodríguez, I; Astola, A; Ortiz, M; Yen, TJ; Bennani, M; Valdivia, MM. Anti-CENPI autoantibodies in scleroderma patients with features of autoimmune liver diseases. *Clin Chim Acta*, 2011, 412, 2267-2271.

In: Scleroderma   ISBN: 978-1-62618-802-0
Editor: Romain De Winter   © 2013 Nova Science Publishers, Inc.

Chapter VI

Iloprost in the Treatment of Raynaud Phenomenon Secondary to Scleroderma

Rebeca Iglesias Barreira[*1], *Hortensia Álvarez Díaz*[2],
Belén Bardán García and Isaura Rodríguez Penín[1]
[1]Department of Pharmacy, Ferrol Health District, Spain
[2]Department of Internal Medicine, Ferrol Health District, Spain

Abstract

Objective: To highlight iloprost as a choice drug in the Raynaud phenomenon secondary to systemic sclerosis, and to forewarn people about the development of a possible paradoxical reaction when repeated intravenous cycles are received.

Background: Raynaud phenomenon occurs in more than 90% of patients with systemic sclerosis. Digital arteries and precapillary arterioles show marked fibrosis of the intima and luminal narrowing, being associated with platelet activation and abnormal vascular reactivity. Iloprost is a prostacyclin analog with vasodilating and platelet inhibitory effects, providing increased blood flow.

[*] Correspondence: Rebeca Iglesias Barreira: rebeca_ib@sefh.es, Address: Avda. de la Residencia s/n., Telephone number: +34981334533 Fax number: +34981334503.

Discussion: The intravenous prostanoids (particularly short-term intravenous infusions of iloprost) have proved to be efficacious in healing digital ulcers and severe Raynaud phenomenon in patients with systemic sclerosis (strength of European League against Rheumatism Scleroderma Trials and Research group- EUSTAR- recommendation A). However, paradoxical reaction of Raynaud phenomenon has been reported in a patient with diffuse cutaneous systemic sclerosis, associated with repeated administration and increased infusion rate of iloprost (probable relationship according to Naranjo probability scale).

Conclusions: Iloprost in treatment of patients with Raynaud phenomenon could be involved in a paradoxical reaction. Physicians should be aware of this adverse event and patients should be monitored (tolerance and clinical response).

Keywords: Systemic sclerosis, Raynaud phenomenon, paradoxical reaction, iloprost

Introduction

Raynaud phenomenon (RP) is extremely common in scleroderma (up to 90% of patients) and often severe [1].

RP is defined as vasospasm of arteries or arterioles causing pallor and at least another colour change upon reperfusion such as cyanosis or redness [1,2,3]. RP occurs as a result of vasoconstriction of the digital arteries, precapillary arterioles, and cutaneous arteriovenous shunts. The initial white phase is marked by demarcated pale skin caused by vasoconstriction and cessation of regional blood flow. The second one is a cyanotic phase as the residual blood in the fingers desaturates. The attack usually ends with rapid reflow of blood to the digits, which results in a red appearance of them. The episode is often accompanied by pain or paresthesia due to sensory nerve ischemia [3,4].

RP can be classified as:

– Primary or idiopathic (Raynaud disease): RP occurs in the absence of causes such as connective tissue disease.
– Secondary: RP occurs in people underlying diseases that affect blood vessels, especially scleroderma and lupus [1,2,3].

The RP that occurs on scleroderma is often more severe in that there is not only vasospasm but also a fixed blood vessel deficit with intimal proliferation and therefore narrowing of the blood vessels. RP may also be accompanied by digital ulcers which are possibly secondary to ischemia due to a vasculopathy characterized histologically by abnormal vascular endothelium and intimal thickening, and clinically by vasospasm [1,5].

It seems that RP that is secondary to scleroderma is not as easily treated as idiopathic RP and it is likely due to the fact that there is underlying obstruction of flow in the blood vessels [1].

Calcium channel antagonists continue to be the drug of choice (strength of recommendation A). However, when RP is severe and is accompanied by digital ulcers/tissue necrosis, the therapeutic regimen must be individualized and combinations should be established with different drugs such as prostanoids, endothelin receptor antagonists such as bosentan, cGMP- specific phosphodiesterase type 5 inhibitor such as sildenafil, antiaggregants /anticoagulants, antibiotics and analgesics [3].

We are going to highlight iloprost as a choice drug in severe Raynaud phenomenon secondary to scleroderma.

Clinical Usefulness of Iloprost in the Treatment of Raynaud Phenomenon

The literature reveals that many different classes of drugs have been demonstrated to have some degree of efficacy in the treatment of RP with respect to decreasing RP frequency and severity, and preventing and healing digital ulcers. Specifically, intravenous iloprost was reported to be effective in the treatment of RP secondary to scleroderma – decreasing the frequency and severity of attacks and preventing or healing digital ulcers [1].

The European League against Rheumatism (EULAR) and the EULAR Scleroderma Trials and Research group (EUSTAR) have developed evidence-based recommendations to be used in clinical practice for the treatment of scleroderma [6].

As stated in these recommendations, intravenous iloprost is a drug that plays an important role in the treatment of RP (strength of recommendation A). Iloprost is a stable analogue of prostacyclin with vasodilating, antiplatelet, cytoprotective, and immunomodulating properties at the systemic and pulmonary levels [6,7].

Iloprost reduces the duration, frequency and severity of scleroderma-related Raynaud phenomenon (SSc-RP) attacks and it should be considered for severe SSc-RP or when dihydropiridine-type calcium antagonists (usually oral nifedipine, and considered first-line therapy for SSc-RP) have failed. Oral prostanoids seem to be generally less effective than intravenous iloprost in the treatment of SSc-RP, although some beneficial effects could be seen with higher doses. Iloprost is only slightly superior to nifedipine in improving symptoms of SSc-RP [4,6].

Furthermore, intravenous prostanoids (in particular iloprost) should be considered in the treatment of active digital ulcers in patients with SSc, as they were shown to improve the healing of active digital ulcers, including ischemic ones [5,6]. The benefit of iloprost on tissue healing may be explained in part by the potential capacity of prostacyclin to inhibit platelet activation and leukocyte adherence to the endothelium, thus reducing counteracting defective endothelial function and tissue injury [5].

Posology and Method of Administration

In the treatment of RP, iloprost is administered in cycles of 3-5 consecutive days, for 6 hours daily via a peripheral vein or a central venous catheter after dilution as an intravenous infusion. The dose of iloprost is adjusted depending on individual tolerance within the range of 0.5 to 2.0 ng of iloprost/kg body weight/min.

The dose tolerated by the patient must be established during the first 2 to 3 days. To this end, the treatment should be initiated at an infusion rate of 0.5 ng/kg/min for 30 minutes. Then the dosage should be increased by 0.5 ng/kg/min at intervals of about every 30 minutes, reaching 2.0 ng/kg/min. Blood pressure and heart rate at the start of the infusion and after each dose increase, and they should be measured. The infusion rate should be accurately calculated based on body weight so that it is within the range 0.5-2.0 ng/kg/min (for use with an infusion pump or an injector). If side effects appear (such as headache and nausea, or an unwanted drop in blood pressure) the infusion rate must be reduced to establish the tolerated dose. If the side effects are severe, the infusion must be discontinued [8].

Undesirable Effects

The pharmacologic action of iloprost is reflected in very common adverse reactions, such as headache (68.8%), flushing due to vasodilation (58.0%), and gastrointestinal symptoms (nausea, diarrhea, vomiting) (up to 29.7%). These are expected to occur at the start of treatment, while adjusting the dose to identify the best tolerance level for each patient [6]. However, all these adverse effects usually disappear rapidly when tapering down the dose. Other related adverse effects are local reactions at the infusion site, such as redness and pain or cutaneous vasodilation [9-14].

A paradoxical reaction of Raynaud phenomenon has been reported in a patient with diffuse cutaneous systemic sclerosis (scleroderma). This adverse reaction was associated with repeated administration and an increased infusion rate of iloprost. In this patient, after the administration of nine cycles of iloprost infusion at a rate from 0.5 ng/kg/min to 1ng/kg/min during five days of every 6-8 weeks, the patient experimented a clear RP in the hand with the infusion line when the rate was increased to 1 ng/kg/min. This happened twice, in cycle numbers ten and eleven; in both cycles, treatment had to be stopped in order to allow his hand to return to a normal temperature and appearance. Due to the lack of therapeutic alternatives, treatment continued at a rate of 0.5 ng/kg/min, which the patient tolerated well, although a cold sensation in the hand with perfusion developed when the infusion rate was increased during both cycles 12 and 13. This adverse event was classified as a probable relationship according to the Naranjo probability scale [5,15].

There was another reported case of a paradoxical reaction with iloprost in a patient with primary pulmonary hypertension, whose pulmonary vascular resistance was increased with inhaled iloprost [16].

A possible explanation for these phenomenons could be that iloprost activates the prostacyclin receptor, with a subsequent rise in intracellular cyclic adenosine monophosphate.

Usually, a rise in cyclic adenosine monophosphate concentrations produces vasodilatation by relaxing smooth muscle cells. In these patients, this cascade may have been altered with the possibility that another prostanoid receptor was activated or that intracellular mechanisms other than those described above were activated [16].

Conclusion

Iloprost may be very effective in the treatment of severe RP secondary to scleroderma. It can reduce the duration, frequency, and severity of RP attacks and increase digital ulcer healing. Iloprost in treatment of patients with Raynaud phenomenon could be involved in a paradoxical reaction, so physicians should be aware of this adverse event and patients should be monitored.

References

[1]   Pope J, Fenlon D, Thomson A, et al. Iloprost and cisaprost for Raynaud's phenomenon in progressive systemic sclerosis. *Cochrane Database of Systematic Reviews 1998, Issue 2.* Art. No.: CD000953. DOI 10.1002/14651858.CD000953.

[2]   Hinchcliff M, Varga J. Systemic sclerosis/scleroderma: a treatable multisystem disease. *Am Fam Physician* 2008; 78:961-8.

[3]   Fonollosa-Pla V, Pilar Simeón-Aznar C, Vilardell-Tarrés M. Treatment of Raynaud's phenomenon. *Rev Clin Esp* 2009;209:21- 4.

[4]   Levien TL. Advances in the treatment of Raynaud's phenomenon.*Vasc Health Risk Manag.* 2010 Mar 24; 6:167-77. PMID:20448801

[5]   Wigley FM, Seibold JR, Wise RA, McCloskey DA, Dole WP. Intravenous iloprost treatment of Raynaud's phenomenon and ischemic ulcers secondary to systemic sclerosis. *J Rheumatol.* 1992; 19:1407–1414.

[6]   Kowal-Bielecka O, Landewe' R, Avouac J, Chwiesko S, Miniati I, et al. EULAR recommendations for the treatment of systemic sclerosis: a report from the EULAR Scleroderma Trials and Research group (EUSTAR)*Ann Rheum Dis* 2009;68:620–628. doi:10.1136/ard.2008. 096677.

[7]   Scorza R, Caronni M, Mascagni B, et al. Effects of long-term cyclic iloprost therapy in systemic sclerosis with Raynaud's phenomenon. A randomized, controlled study. *Clin Exp Rheumatol* 2001;19:503-8.

[8]   Ilomedin data sheet. Madrid: Agencia Española de Medicamentos y Productos Sanitarios, 2010-2011. *https://sinaem4.agemed.es/consaem/ especialidad.*do?metodo=verFichaWordPdf&codigo=61596&formato=p df&formulario=FICHAS&file=ficha.pdf (accessed 2013 Jan 11).

[9]   McHugh NJ, Csuka M, Watson H, et al. Infusion of iloprost, a prostacyclin analogue, for treatment of Raynaud's phenomenon in systemic sclerosis.*Ann Rheum Dis* 1988;47:43-7.

[10] Black CM, Halkier-Sorensen L, Belch JJ, et al. Oral iloprost in Raynaud'sphenomenon secondary to systemic sclerosis: a multicentre, placebo-controlled,dose-comparison study. *Br J Rheumatol* 1998; 37: 952-60.

[11] Kawald A, Burmester GR, Huscher D, Sunderkötter C, Riemekasten G.Low versus high-dose iloprost therapy over 21 days in patients with secondary Raynaud's phenomenon and systemic sclerosis: a randomized,open, single-center study. *J Rheumatol* 2008; 35: 1830-7.

[12] Marasini B, Massarotti M, Bottaso B, et al. Comparison between iloprost and alprostadil in the treatment of Raynaud's phenomenon. *Scand J Rheumatol* 2004; 33:253-6.

[13] Wigley FM, Wise RA, Seibold JR, et al. Intravenous iloprost infusion inpatients with Raynaud phenomenon secondary to systemic sclerosis. A multicenter, placebo-controlled, double-blind study. *Ann Intern Med* 1994; 120: 199-206.

[14] Torley HI, Madhok R, Capell HA, et al. A double blind, randomised, multicentre comparison of two doses of intravenous iloprost in the treatment of Raynaud's phenomenon secondary to connective tissue diseases. *Ann Rheum Dis* 1991; 50: 800- 4.

[15] Barreira RI, García BB, López MG, Legazpi IR, Díaz HÁ, Penín IR. Paradoxical reaction of raynaud phenomenon following the repeated administration of iloprost in a patient with diffuse cutaneous systemic sclerosis. *Ann Pharmacother.* 2012 Oct; 46(10):e28. doi: 10.1345/aph. 1R093. Epub 2012 Oct 2.

[16] Emmel M, Keuth B, Schickendantz S. Paradoxical increase of pulmonary vascular resistance during testing of inhaled iloprost. *Heart* 2004; 90:e2.

Index

U

V

W

X

Y